# Color Atlas of
# Diagnostic
# Microbiology

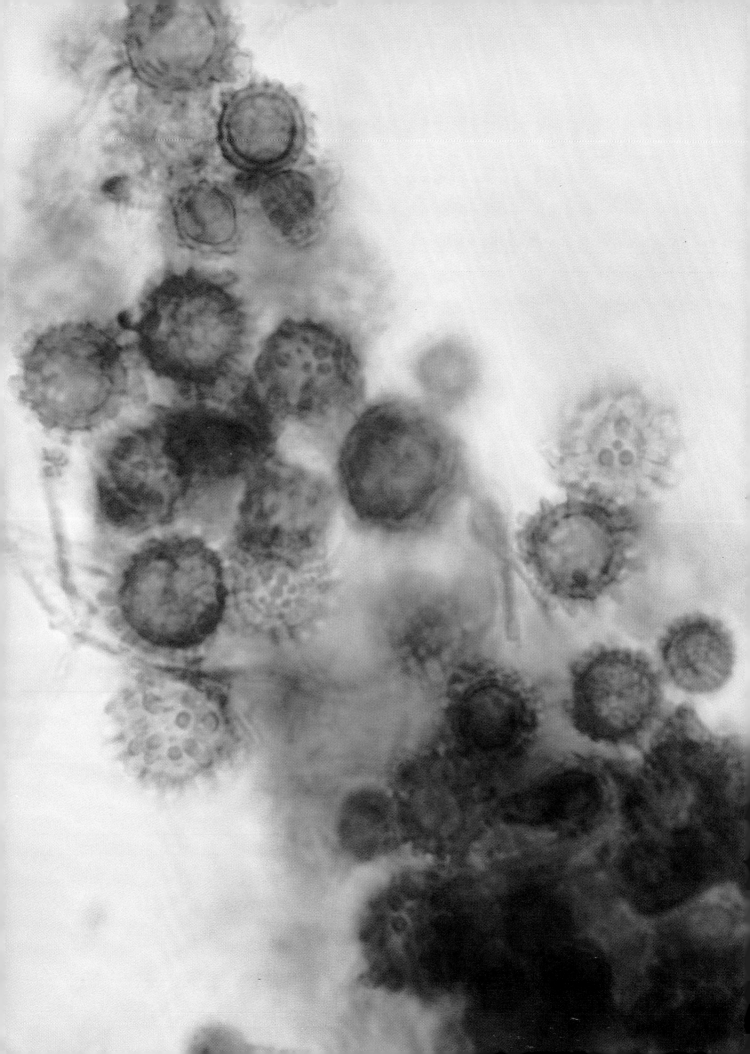

# Color Atlas of Diagnostic Microbiology

*Luis M. de la Maza, M.D., Ph.D.*
Professor, Department of Pathology
Director, Division of Medical Microbiology
University of California, Irvine Medical Center
Orange, California

*Marie T. Pezzlo, M.A., F(AAM)*
Administrative Director
Department of Pathology
University of California, Irvine Medical Center
Orange, California

*Ellen Jo Baron, Ph.D., F(AAM)*
Adjunct Associate Professor of Medicine
University of California, Los Angeles
Clinical Associate Professor of Molecular Microbiology and Immunology
University of Southern California
Los Angeles, California

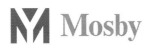 Mosby

St. Louis  Baltimore  Boston  Carlsbad  Chicago  Naples  New York  Philadelphia  Portland
London  Madrid  Mexico City  Singapore  Sydney  Tokyo  Toronto  Wiesbaden

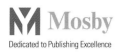
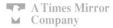

*Vice President/Publisher:* Don Ladig
*Editor:* Jennifer Roche
*Developmental Editor:* Sandra J. Parker
*Project Manager:* Linda McKinley
*Production Editor:* Rich Barber
*Designer:* Elizabeth Fett
*Manufacturing Supervisor:* Theresa Fuchs

Printed in the United States of America
Composition and Lithography/color film by GTS Graphics
Printing/binding by Walsworth Press, Inc.

Mosby-Year Book, Inc.
11830 Westline Industrial Drive
St. Louis, Missouri 63146

**International Standard Book Number**
0-8151-0621-1

97  98  99  00  01  /  9  8  7  6  5  4  3  2  1

# Preface

Infectious diseases caused more than 17 million deaths in 1995, almost one third of all deaths that occurred worldwide that year. The World Health Organization has listed 18 "new" infectious diseases identified during the last 22 years that are contributing to these statistics. This ominous rise in infectious diseases is accompanied by an almost equally alarming decrease in the numbers of programs available for training clinical laboratory scientists and microbiologists.

Diagnostic microbiology is a visual science; ability to recognize characteristics both microscopically and macroscopically is the hallmark of competence in the field. A convenient and inclusive source of microbiological color images is virtually nonexistent. We have sought to remedy that situation with this volume.

The book contains 753 full-color images, encompassing laboratory safety practices, specimen collection and transport devices, specimen handling, colony morphologies, microscopic images, biochemicals and other tests, and susceptibility testing. The microbes that cause human disease are found among viruses, fungi, parasites, and bacteria, and this book includes representative images from each group. Emphasis has been placed on the pictures and text is minimal, with just enough information to place the photographs into context. The book is meant to be a collection of some of the most important visual images in human diagnostic microbiology.

All instructors helping students to learn medical microbiology know how difficult it is sometimes to find that "typical" image to illustrate a point. We expect this book will provide instructors easy access to those images that are frequently used in the teaching of diagnostic microbiology. The book should be useful to medical students taking their microbiology courses, pathology residents and infectious diseases fellows, pathologists and physicians, and of course, laboratory scientists and diagnostic microbiologists, both beginning and reviewing.

We have attempted to include in this atlas those images that cover the most frequently detected pathogens and most frequently performed tests in the clinical laboratory. We realize that this is an impossible task, because the numbers of pathogens and types of tests vary greatly from site to site. If we have failed to cover a subject that you think should be included, please feel free to send us your suggestions, or even better, specimens and samples, to be considered for the next edition of this book. Obviously, we ask all of our readers, and particularly our critics, to bring to our attention any errors that they may find in the book. We thank all of you in advance for your help.

## Technical Note

The light and fluorescent microscopic pictures were taken with a Zeiss Universal microscope (Carl Zeiss Inc., West Germany) equipped with Zeiss and Olympus (Olympus Optical Corp., Ltd., Japan) lenses, and a Nikon FX-35A camera (Nikon Corp., Tokyo, Japan). The macroscopic images were obtained using a Nikon EL camera with a Micro-Nikkor 55 mm f/3.5 lens, and a Contax RTS camera with a Carl Zeiss S-Planar 60 mm f/2.8 lens. Kodachrome 25 Professional film (Eastman Kodak Co., Rochester, New York) and Velvia and Provia Fujichrome films (Fuji Photo Film Co., Ltd., Tokyo, Japan) were used for most of the images. The electron micrographs were taken with a Philips EM400 electron microscope (Philips Electronic Instruments Co., Eindhoven, The Netherlands) and Electron Image Film SO-163 (Eastman Kodak Co.). The magnification stated in the legends corresponds to approximately that of the printed figure. However, for calculation, the measurement provided in the legend should be used.

## Acknowledgments

Special thanks for their extra effort go to all the staff of the Division of Medical Microbiology at UCI Medical Center. We are especially grateful to Sandra Aarnaes, Jeanne Blanding, Megan Codd, Neil Detweiler, Kaye Evans, Janet Shigei, Radha Srikumar, Grace Tan, and Minas Zartarian for their help in preparing the specimens and collecting the material for inclusion in this book.

*This book is dedicated to all past and present members of the staff of the Division of Medical Microbiology at UCI Medical Center. Their commitment to patient care and teaching made this book possible. And to* Frank Pezzlo *and* James C. Taylor *for their unending support.*

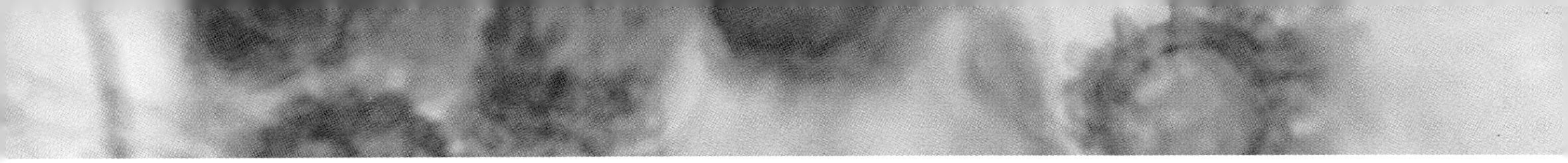

# Contents

1 Laboratory Safety, 1

2 Specimen Collection Containers, 9

3 Specimen Processing, 14

4 Gram Stain, 25

5 Micrococcaceae, 32

6 Streptococcaceae, 37

7 Aerobic Gram-Positive Bacilli & Actinomyces spp., 46

8 Enterobacteriaceae, 56

9 Other Gram-Negative Microorganisms, 72

10 Anaerobic Bacteria, 88

11 Mycobacteria, 95

12 Microbial Pathogens Isolated and/or Identified by Tissue Culture or Other
   Special Methods, 102

13 Antimicrobial Susceptibility Testing, 107

14 Mycology, 113

15 Parasitology, 146

16 Virology, 176

17 Immunoserology, 194

18 Molecular Techniques, 200

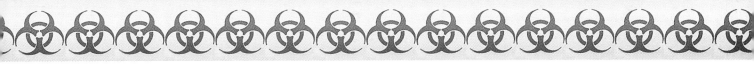

# CHAPTER 1 *Laboratory Safety*

During the last decade there has been a dramatic increase in the number of guidelines, recommendations, regulations, and standards introduced for the safety of personnel working with potential pathogens in clinical laboratories. It is mandated by OSHA (Occupational Safety and Health Act, created 1970) that guidelines be implemented and practiced and that protective clothing, containment devices, and decontamination equipment and materials be available in the workplace. Procedures regarding biosafety requirements and practices must be available and familiar to all laboratory personnel.

## Protective Clothing and Equipment

An important component of Universal Precautions and safe work practices is the effective use of protective gloves, eye and mouth protection, and laboratory coats, all considered to be Personal Protective Devices. Protective gloves must be worn whenever there is a potential for direct contact with infectious materials. Disposable latex or vinyl gloves are recommended and should immediately be discarded in a designated waste container when removed.

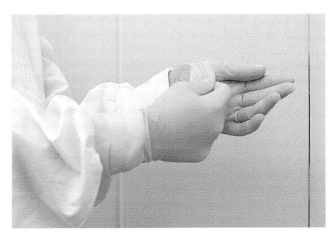

**1-1** Remove one glove by pulling the outside bottom of that glove toward the palm and fingers with the other gloved hand, turning the glove inside out as it is removed. Do not touch your skin with the outer glove surface.

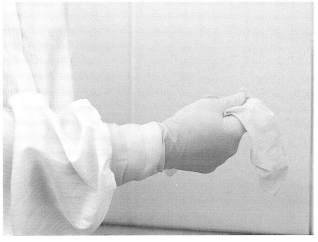

**1-2** Pull the glove completely off and hold this contaminated glove in the gloved hand. Do not touch the outer surface of either glove with the ungloved hand.

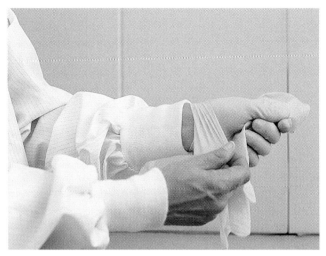

**1-3** Using the ungloved hand, grab the inside of the bottom of the second glove and pull the other glove off.

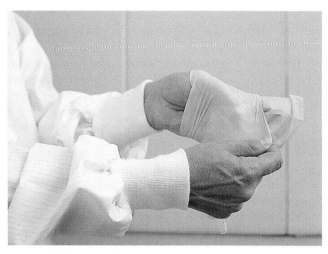

**1-4** Pull the second glove over the contaminated glove that is held in the hand, turning it completely inside out to contain the first glove and to avoid contaminating the ungloved hands.

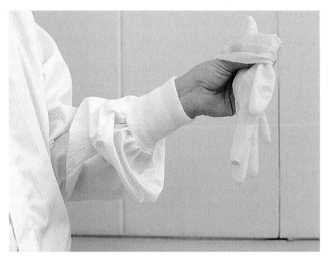

**1-5** Both gloves should be immediately discarded in a waste container designated for contaminated materials.

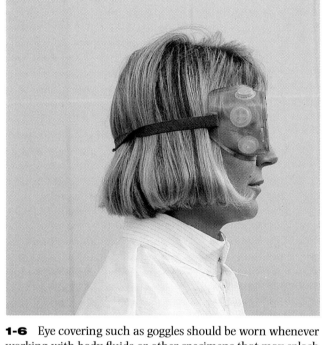

**1-6** Eye covering such as goggles should be worn whenever working with body fluids or other specimens that may splash or procedures that may create aerosols. Goggles with side panels should be provided for each worker.

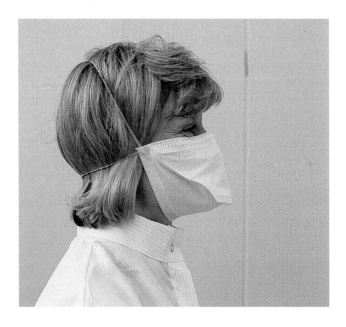

**1-7** A face mask is worn to protect mucous membranes of the nose and mouth and to screen out aerosol particles that may enter the respiratory or digestive tracts. The mask should fit tightly around the face and provide the OSHA-mandated level of protection. Face masks should always be worn if there is a chance of spattering clinical material. In some settings, waterproof face shields may be required for some tasks involving serum and blood.

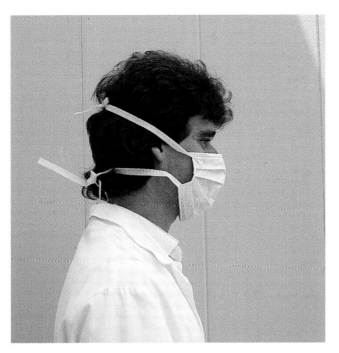

**1-8** This photograph illustrates an improperly fitted face mask that does not provide adequate protection. There is a potential for contaminated materials to enter through the gaps and come into contact with mucous membranes or to be breathed in.

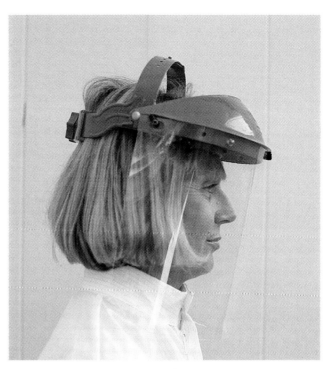

**1-9** A full face shield protects the eyes, nose, and mouth.

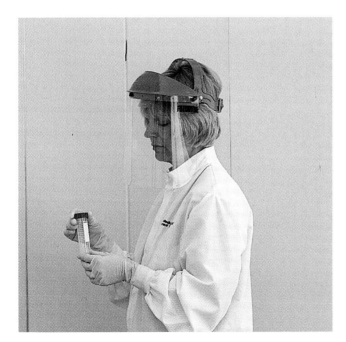

**1-10** A full face shield is worn to protect the eyes, nose, and mouth from splashes.

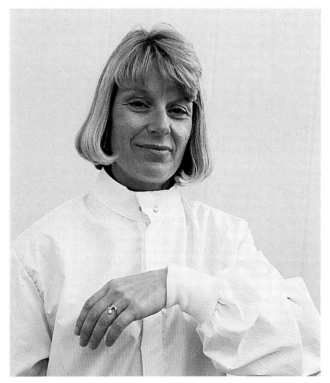

**1-11** Fluid-resistant laboratory coats with closed necks and wrists should be worn to cover all potential exposed skin and clothing. Fluid-resistant laboratory coats should be worn over street clothes and should be removed before leaving the laboratory.

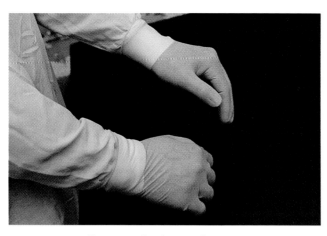

**1-12**   Knit cuffs protect the skin on the arms.

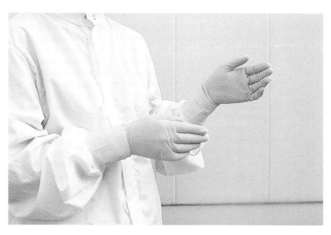

**1-13**   Protective gloves should be worn over the knit cuffs to provide a proper sleeve closure and hand protection.

# Disinfection, Waste Disposal, and Sterilization

## Disinfection

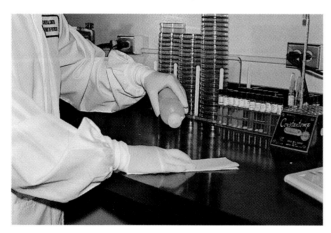

**1-14**   Decontamination of work surfaces at the end of each shift and cleaning of spills should be performed with a fresh 10% solution of household bleach.

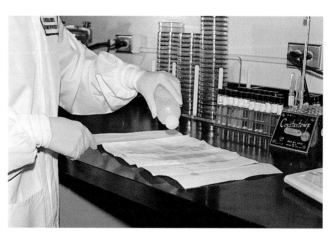

**1-15**   Paper towels should be placed on the contaminated work surface and soaked with diluted household bleach immediately after a spill and at the end of each shift.

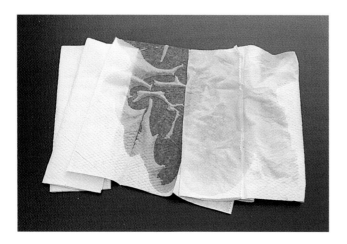

**1-16**   Bleach-soaked paper towels should also be used in the biological safety cabinet to catch fallen drops that can create aerosols.

## Waste Disposal

Contaminated materials should be disposed of in proper containers that are properly labeled and fitted with lids. Separate containers are available for plastic and glass and needles. It is important to dispose of materials in proper containers to avoid potentially serious injury or illness to individuals coming in contact with these materials.

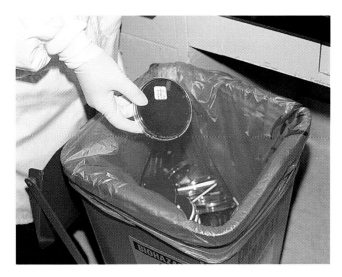

**1-17** Agar plates are discarded in a properly labeled container with a lid.

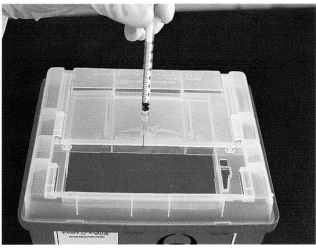

**1-18** Needles with attached syringes are discarded into hard-sided, puncture-proof containers. Needles must never be recapped unless a specially designed, commercially available holder for resheathing needles is used for that purpose.

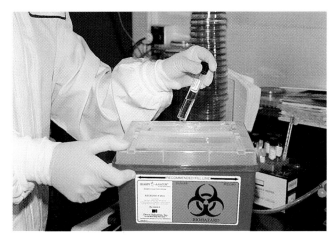

**1-19** Glass tubes containing human samples are also discarded into hard-sided, puncture-proof containers.

## Sterilization

All materials contaminated with potentially infectious microorganisms must be decontaminated before disposal. An autoclave is the most common instrument used to perform this function.

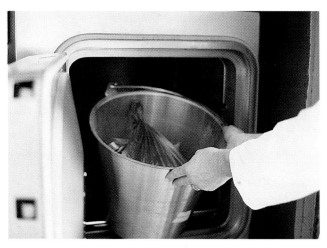

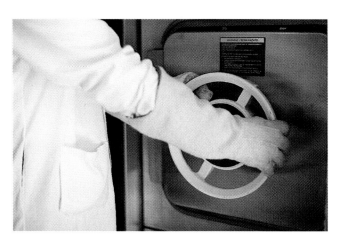

**1-20**  Loosely packed materials that have been appropriately discarded in designated containers (i.e., red-bagged lined buckets, are placed in the autoclave). The bags, which should never be filled completely, are loosely tied at the top to allow the steam to circulate and effectively decontaminate the contents. Adding approximately 1 cup of water to the bag facilitates steam production.

**1-21**  The autoclave door is closed tightly. At the completion of the cycle, the door is opened slowly by an operator wearing heat-resistant gloves and a face mask to protect against burns from escaping steam.

## Biological Safety Cabinet

The biological safety cabinet (BSC) is one of the most common containment devices used in laboratories. Air is decontaminated by high-efficiency particulate air (HEPA) filters.

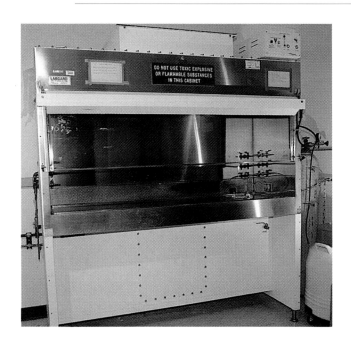

**1-22**  A commonly used Class II biological safety cabinet that filter sterilizes both the incoming and exhausted air. A BSC should be kept free of clutter. Routine inspection of the cabinet by a certified technician is required.

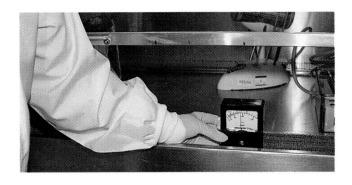

**1-23** Regular measuring of air flow should be performed to ensure proper velocity. Mechanical problems, filter clogging, and other reasons contribute to lowered velocity, which may allow infectious particles to escape the cabinet.

## Other Safety Practices

Use of aerosol-containing safety buckets in centrifuges, vortexing tightly sealed tubes in a biological safety cabinet (BSC), and securing gas tanks to a holding device mounted on the wall are other additional safety practices that are required to ensure a safe work environment.

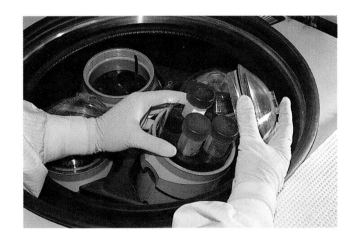

**1-24** Tightly sealed centrifuge tubes are placed into safety carriers that are themselves tightly sealed before centrifugation. This will avoid creating an aerosol if tubes are broken during centrifugation.

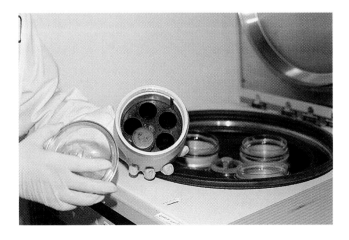

**1-25** Care should be taken when opening a sealed centrifuge carrier to avoid contamination from a possible broken container during centrifugation.

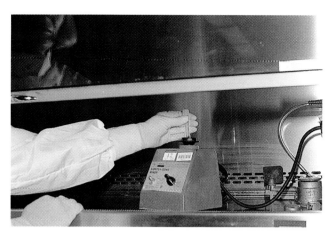

**1-26**   Tightly sealed containers should be vortexed in a BSC only. The tube should then be inverted to reabsorb aerosolized particles. A 30-minute wait before opening the tube avoids aerosol creation, especially when mycobacteria are being handled.

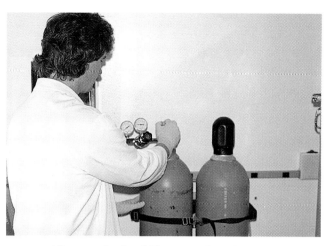

**1-27**   All gas tanks should be secured in place by a holding device.

## Mailing Containers

Potentially infectious material must be shipped according to the federal codes of Interstate Shipment of Etiologic Agents.

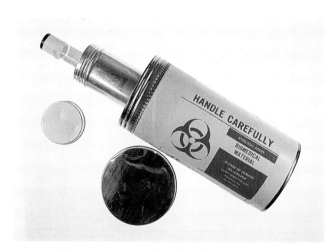

**1-28**   The specimen must be placed in an inner sealed container, which is then placed in an outer sealed metal tube. The inner container must have sufficient material to absorb the entire fluid contents in the event of a leak.

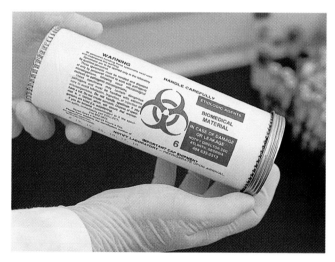

**1-29**   An official *Etiologic Agents* label must be affixed to the outer container.

# CHAPTER 2 *Specimen Collection Containers*

**I**t is the responsibility of the diagnostic microbiology laboratory to select and provide transport devices for collection of specimens from a variety of anatomical sites. Most specimen collection containers incorporate transport media that support the viability of microorganisms encountered in clinical specimens. The interpretation of results is dependent upon the quality of the collected specimen and the transport conditions. Improperly transported specimens may result in failure to isolate the causative microorganism. One of the most common and widely used transport systems is a plastic tube containing a sterile polyester-tipped swab and medium to prevent the drying of microorganisms, maintain the pH, and minimize overgrowth.

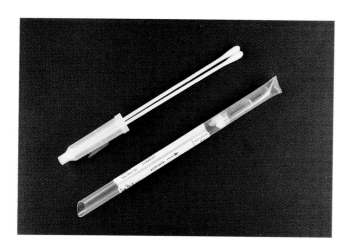

**2-1 Sterile disposable aerobic culture collection and transport system** consisting of a plastic tube containing two rayon-tipped swabs and modified Stuart's transport medium in a separate ampoule (BBL Microbiology Systems, Cockeysville, Md.). The ampoule is located at the base of the tube and is covered by a protective sleeve on the outside. This ampoule must be crushed after the specimen is collected, and the swabs are placed back into the container to keep the specimen on the swabs moist. The use of cotton swabs should be avoided because they contain fatty acids that may be inhibitory to some bacteria.

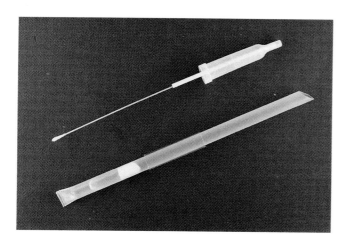

**2-2 Nasopharyngeal-urogenital swab (Calgiswab Type IV; Spectrum Diagnostics, Glenwood, Ill.).** This flexible wire shaft and small tip provides easy specimen collection, especially for nasopharyngeal and male urethral specimens. Calcium alginate swabs should not be used for collection of urethral specimens because they can be toxic to some strains of *Neisseria gonorrhoeae*; however, they are useful for collection of *Chlamydia trachomatis* cultures.

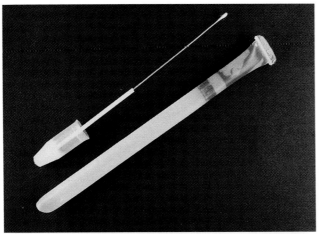

**2-3 Nasopharyngeal collection system.** A similar collection system as described in Figure 2-2; however, this swab is used for collection of nasopharyngeal specimens for recovery of *Bordetella pertussis*. The tube contains Amies' charcoal transport medium, which also supports the viability of *Neisseria gonorrhoeae*.

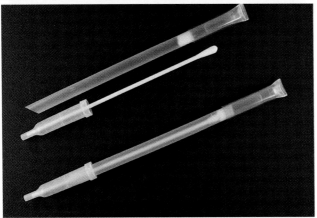

**2-4 Sterile, disposable collection and transport system for recovery of viruses (BBL Microbiology Systems, Cockeysville, Md.).** The swab and holder are shown separately at the top and assembled at the bottom. The tube contains a rayon-tipped swab and viral transport medium containing Hanks' balanced salt solution and antimicrobics. This prevents specimen drying, helps maintain viral viability, and retards the growth of other microbial contaminants.

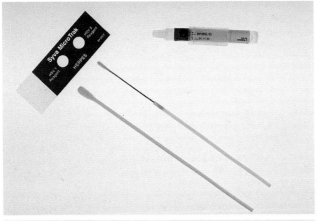

**2-5 Herpes collection kit** containing two sizes of dacron-tipped swabs, a slide for preparation of a direct smear at the time of collection, and a slide fixative (Syva MicroTrak, San Jose, Calif.). The slide will be stained later in the laboratory with a direct fluorescent antibody stain.

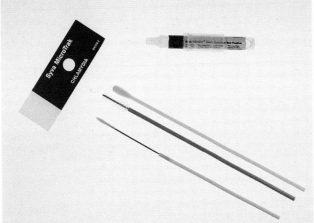

**2-6 *Chlamydia trachomatis* collection kit** containing two sizes of dacron-tipped swabs and a cytobrush, a slide for preparation of a direct smear at the time of collection, and an ampoule of slide fixative (Syva MicroTrak, San Jose, Calif.). The slide will be stained later in the laboratory with a direct fluorescent antibody stain.

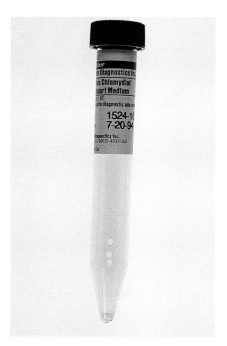

**2-7 Viral-chlamydial transport medium.** Specimens for detection of viruses or chlamydia should be placed into a tube of sucrose-phosphate buffer transport medium containing fetal calf serum, buffer, and gentamicin (Baxter Diagnostics, Inc., Deerfield, Ill.).

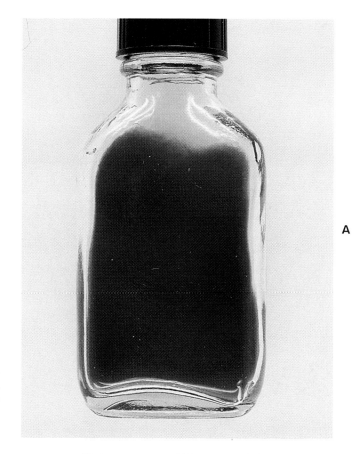

A

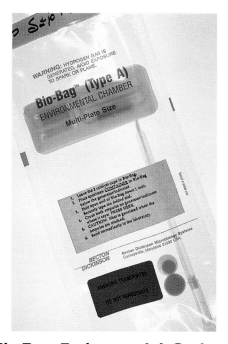

**2-8 Bio-Bag Environmental System (BBL Microbiology Systems, Cockeysville, Md.).** The specimen for anaerobic culture is collected as tissue in a sterile tube or, much less desirable, on a swab, and then placed in the gas impermeable environmental bag that contains ampoules of indicator, catalyst, and hydrogen-$CO_2$ generator. The bag is sealed and each ampoule is crushed to produce anaerobic conditions.

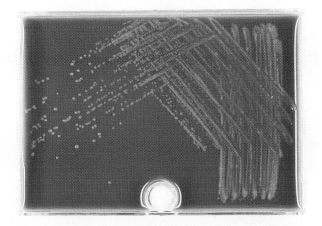

B

**2-9 A, Transgrow bottle (BBL Microbiology Systems, Cockeysville, Md.)** for recovery of *Neisseria gonorrhoeae.* The inner flat surface of the bottle contains modified Thayer-Martin agar that has been prepared under $CO_2$. **B, Jembec plate (BBL Microbiology Systems, Cockeysville, Md.)** for recovery of *Neisseria gonorrhoeae.* Medium is prepared in a flat, plastic container with a snap-top lid. The specimen is inoculated directly, and the moisture from the medium dissolves a bicarbonate tablet to create the $CO_2$ atmosphere.

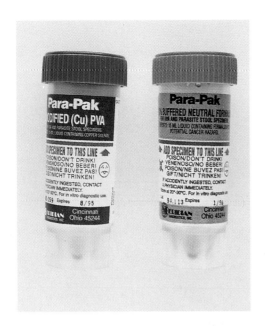

**2-10 Para-Pak Parasitology Collection Kit (Meridian Diagnostics, Cincinnati, Ohio).** This commercially prepared kit contains one vial of modified polyvinyl alcohol (PVA) and one vial of buffered neutral formalin. Placing the stool specimen into these vials immediately after collection preserves the morphology of the parasites.

There are a variety of media for the collection and recovery of microorganisms from blood. Some of these media can be used alone, while others require incubation and detection in an automated system. They all contain between 0.025% to 0.05% sodium polyanetholsulfonate (SPS), and the recommended blood-to-medium ratio is 1:2.5 to 1:10, depending upon the system. Examples of these media appear in Figures 2-11 to 2-14.

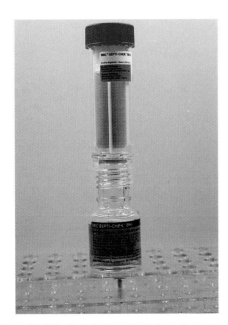

**2-11 Septi-Chek biphasic blood culture bottle (BBL Microbiology Systems, Cockeysville, Md.)** represents a nonautomated blood culture system. Bottles contain tryptic soy broth and an agar slide paddle with three agar types: chocolate, MacConkey, and malt. Blood is inoculated into the bottle at the time of collection and transported to the laboratory. In a biological safety cabinet, an agar slide paddle is attached to the bottle, inverted, and incubated. Subcultures are performed by inverting the bottle again to inoculate the paddle.

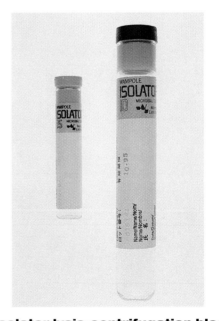

**2-12 Isolator lysis-centrifugation blood culture system, 1.5 and 10-ml tubes (Wampole Laboratories, Cranbury, N.J.)** are recommended for the isolation of mycobacteria and fungi. The tube contains a blood cell lysing fluid of saponin, polypropylene, SPS, fluorinert, and EDTA. Specimens collected in the 10-ml tube are centrifuged at 3000 × g for 30 minutes. The supernatant is discarded, and the sediment is plated onto selected media. Specimens collected in the 1.5 ml tube are plated directly onto media.

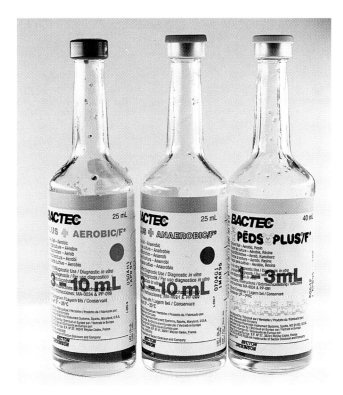

**2-13 BACTEC blood culture bottles** are manufactured with a choice of media, such as 26 Plus, 27 Plus, and Peds Plus, shown here. The bottles are used with the 9000 Fluorescent Series Instrument (BDDIS, Becton Dickinson, Sparks, Md.). These media are intended for recovery of aerobic and anaerobic microorganisms.

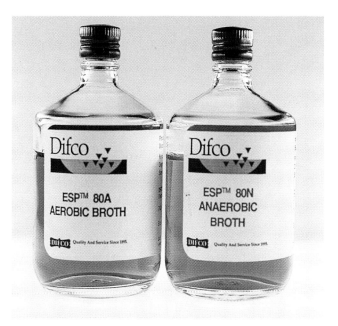

**2-14 ESP 80A aerobic and 80N anaerobic blood culture media** to be used with the ESP automated blood culture system (Difco Laboratories, Detroit, Mich.).

**2-15 Blood collection vacutainer tubes.** Three blood collection vacutainer tubes (*left to right*): SPS-containing, serum separator type, and sodium heparin-containing (Becton Dickinson, Cockeysville, Md.). The plasma or serum obtained is used for the serodiagnosis of infectious diseases.

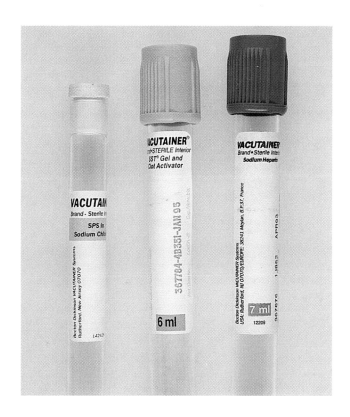

CHAPTER 3 *Specimen Processing*

T here are a number of important steps involved in specimen processing that include (1) entry of patient information into a computer system or manual log; (2) visual examination of the specimen to determine if acceptance criteria are met; (3) specimen preparation, selection, and inoculation of media; and (4) preparation and microscopic examination of direct smears. Upon receipt into the laboratory, the technologist should verify that the specimen is labeled with the appropriate patient information. Unlabeled and mislabeled specimens should be handled according to the written laboratory policy. Any additional patient information needed to process the specimen should be retrieved from the laboratory information system (LIS) or other source.

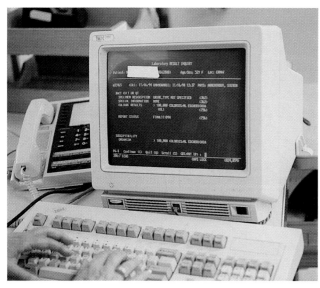

**3-1** Entry of specimen information into the computer system. Upon receipt into the laboratory, the specimen should be entered into the LIS or manual logbook. Patient information including diagnosis and antimicrobial therapy, complete specimen information including anatomic collection site, time of collection, and test requests, and specimen accession number should be available before specimen processing.

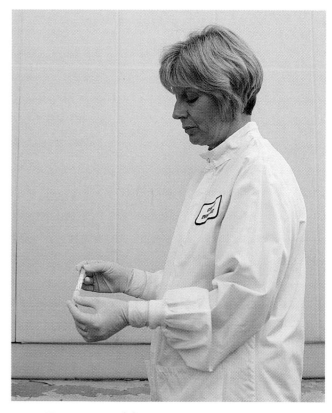

**3-2** Examination of the specimen container to confirm that the specimen is properly labeled, a criterion for acceptance. A protocol for handling unlabeled and mislabeled specimens should be available and followed.

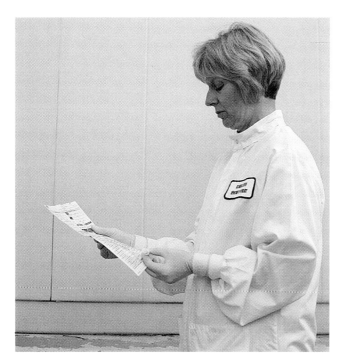

**3-3** Verifying that the information on the specimen container label corresponds with the laboratory request form. Improperly labeled specimens should be processed only if corrective action and documentation are complete.

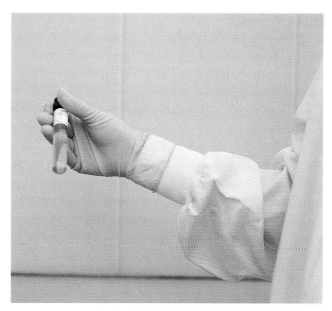

**3-4** Carefully examining the specimen to determine if it matches the specimen description provided on the laboratory request form.

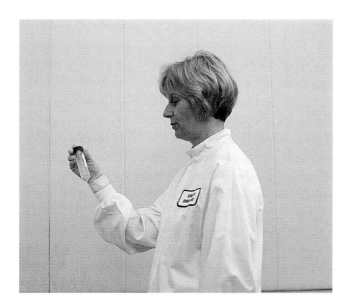

**3-5** Examining the specimen container for the presence of cracks, leaks, and other potential problems. Universal precautions should be used when handling all specimens.

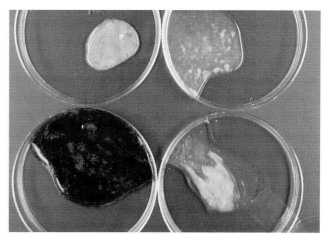

**3-6** Macroscopic examination is an important determination for all specimens; however, it is imperative for specimens from expectorated sputa. The macroscopic appearances of the four sputum specimens shown in this figure are: (*top left*) thick, mucoid, purulent; (*top right*) watery saliva; (*bottom left*) mucoid, bloody; (*bottom left*) thick, mucoid center surrounded by saliva.

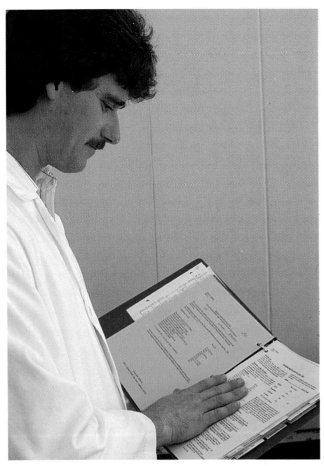

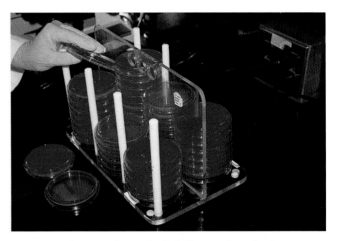

**3-7**   A well-written procedure manual must be available. It should include policies for accepting and rejecting specimens, and guidelines for specimen processing. This manual should be consulted for complete information on specimen processing, inoculation of media, and incubation and atmospheric conditions.

**3-8**   A selection of enriched, differential, and selective media should be available for culture. A daily supply of media should be stored at room temperature and easily accessible to the user.

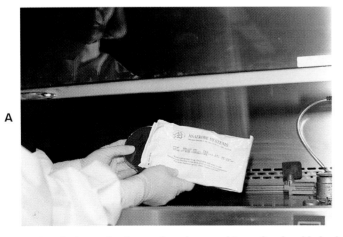

A

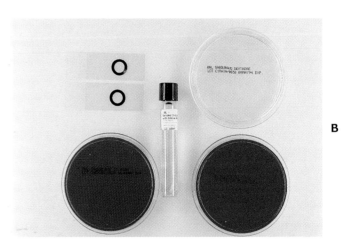

B

**3-9**   **A,** A supply of prereduced anaerobic media should also be available and used only on selected specimens as outlined in the procedure manual. **B,** The appropriate media and slides should be selected on the basis of the specimen source and culture request. These media should be labeled with the patient identifying/accession number before they are inoculated.

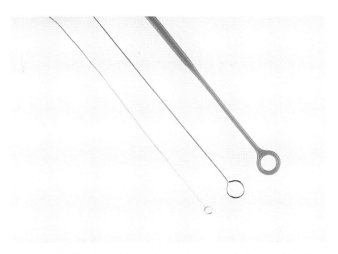

**3-10** A selection of inoculating loops, including calibrating loops, should be among the supplies for processing.

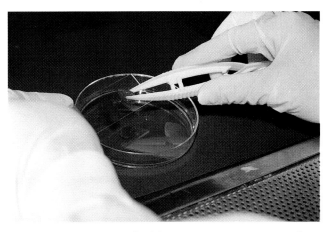

**3-11** An excellent method for preparing a Gram stain from fresh tissue is to press the tissue directly onto the slide surface. Sterile slides should be used to preserve the tissue for additional studies.

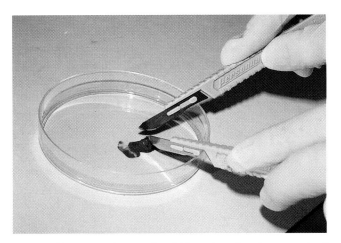

**3-12** Tissue specimens should be minced or homogenized before inoculation onto media. One method makes use of sterile scalpel blades. The specimen is placed into a sterile petri dish, and one or two sterile surgical scalpels are used to mince the specimen until it is homogeneous in consistency.

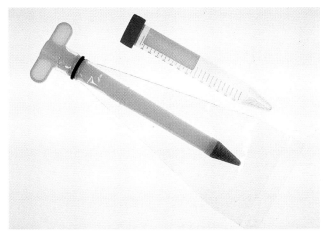

**3-13** Another method for homogenizing tissue is using a disposable tissue-grinding kit (Sage Products, Cary, Ill.). This system minimizes contamination and splattering of the specimen.

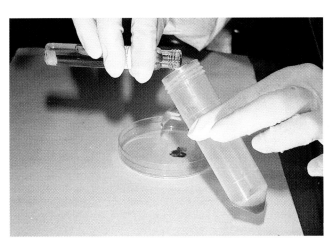

**3-14** A portion of the specimen is placed into the tissue grinder tube, and at least 0.5 ml of nutrient broth is added to moisten the specimen.

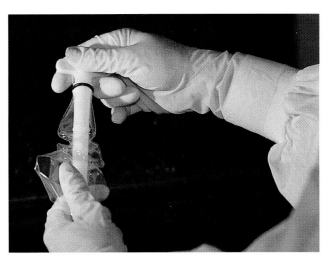

**3-15** The specimen is homogenized as the operator twists and pushes the pestle down onto the tissue. The procedure should always be performed in a biological safety cabinet.

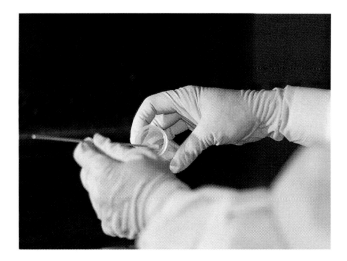

**3-16** Specimens must be examined carefully before inoculation of media. A representative portion that has an abnormal appearance (i.e., flecks of blood, mucous, granules, purulent, abnormal color, or other signs of an infectious process) should be selected.

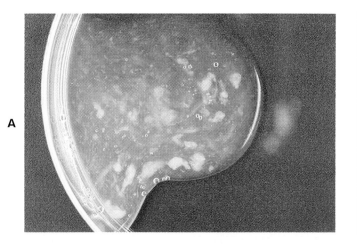

A

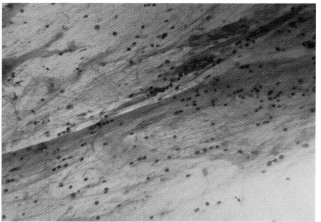

B

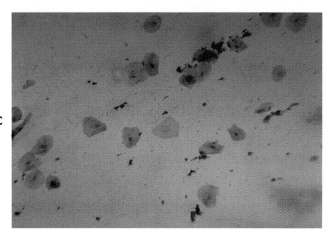

C

**3-17 A,** Saliva, as shown in this figure, must be distinguished from sputum. The impression that a specimen consists of saliva is confirmed by preparing a Gram stain and examining the specimen microscopically. If the microscopic examination confirms that the specimen is not sputum, the specimen should be rejected and not processed for routine bacterial culture. **B,** Gram stain (low power) of a good quality sputum specimen, characterized by lack of squamous epithelial cells. Most of the somatic cells seen are neutrophils. **C,** Gram stain (low power) of a poor quality sputum specimen, characterized by numerous squamous epithelial cells. The culture of such a specimen will not accurately reflect the clinical situation and may yield misleading results.

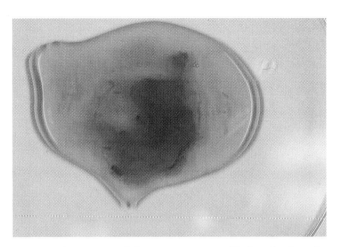

**3-18** The portion of the specimen most likely to harbor the infecting microorganisms is selected. A sample of this sputum specimen should be taken from the central, bloody portion.

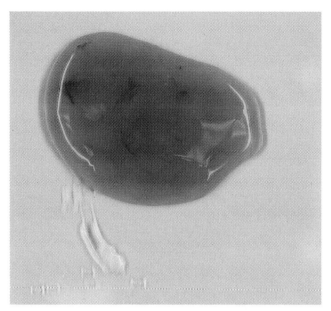

**3-19** Rejection of specimens that appear macroscopically to be from an infected source, such as the exudate fluid shown in this figure, but appear unacceptable when examined microscopically, should be avoided. The Gram stain should be repeated if there is a discrepancy between the microscopic exam and the gross appearance of the specimen.

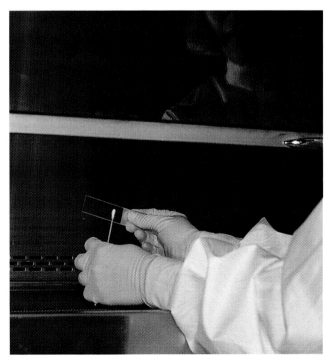

**3-20** Proper technique should be used when preparing direct smears. When inoculating a specimen onto a slide with a swab, the swab should be rolled over most of the surface using a back-and-forth motion. Reject dry swabs and request a new specimen.

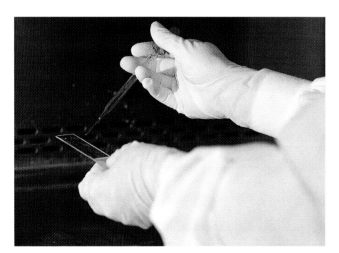

**3-21** When a sterile Pasteur pipette is used to inoculate fluids onto a slide, enough specimen must be placed on the slide to form a circle of approximately 15 mm in diameter. The slide should air dry in the biological safety cabinet before it is fixed and stained.

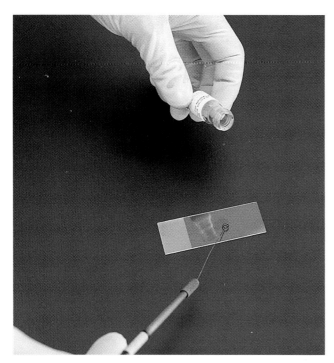

**3-22**  It may be necessary to use a loop to prepare the slide if the sample is small. Enough specimen should be deposited on the slide to form a circle of approximately 15 mm in diameter. Clear fluids, on the other hand, should be deposited in a heaped drop and allowed to air dry. A cytocentrifuge is recommended for making smears of body fluids.

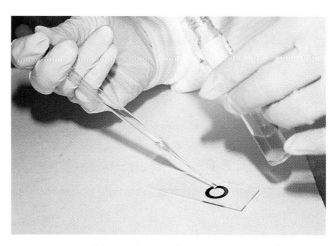

**3-23**  A small drop of a liquid specimen is placed in a well on a slide and covered immediately with a cover slip. This preparation is examined under ×400 power to detect bacterial motility, motile parasites, and for other investigations.

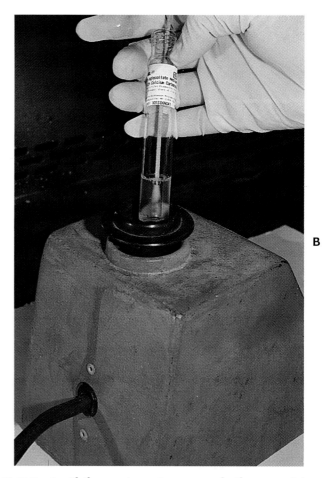

B

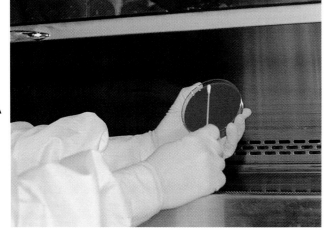

A

**3-24**  **A,** If the specimen is on a swab, the agar plates should be inoculated by rotating the swab across one quadrant of the plate. **B,** If only one swab is available, it should be vortexed in a small amount of broth (0.75 to 1.0 ml) and the resulting suspension can be used to inoculate plates and prepare the smear. Vortexing should be performed in a biological safety cabinet.

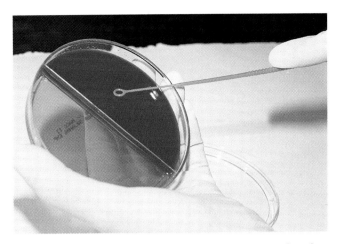

**3-24, cont.**  **C,** The primary inoculum is spread with a loop, using a back-and-forth motion. A wire loop should be sterilized between each successive quadrant streak.

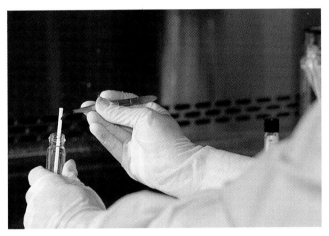

**3-26**  Sterile forceps are used to process hardware such as catheter tips. The forceps are first used to roll the catheter tip over the entire surface of an agar plate, and then to place the catheter tip into a broth medium (shown).

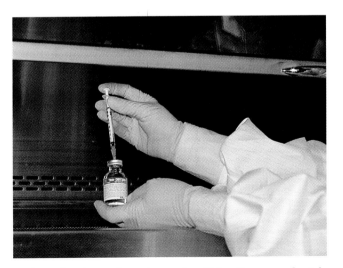

**3-27**  Specimens in syringes should be discouraged; vials are best inoculated at the bedside. Blood culture vials are useful for many body fluids.

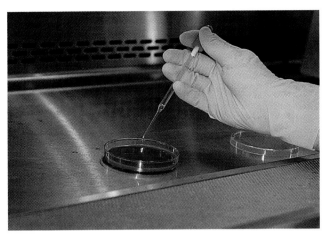

**3-25**  If sterile body fluids are concentrated by centrifugation, the supernatant should be aspirated off the sediment, and a Pasteur pipette should be used to mix and then inoculate the sediment onto media and slides. Volumes too small to be centrifuged should be inoculated directly with a pipette.

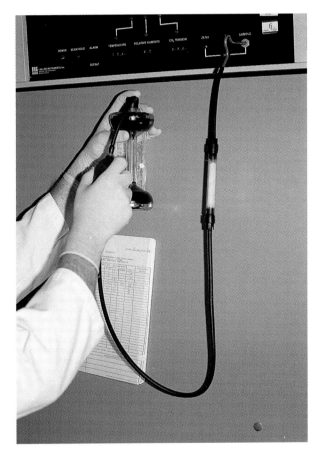

**3-28**  A variety of atmospheric conditions and incubation temperatures should be available for recovery of pathogenic microorganisms. Incubation temperatures should include at least 30°C, 35°C, and 42°C, along with aerobic, anaerobic, capneic, and microaerophilic conditions. Most routine aerobic cultures should be incubated at 35° to 37°C in a humid atmosphere of 5% to 7% $CO_2$. The temperature, $CO_2$ content, and humidity should be monitored daily. The $CO_2$ content is measured with a gauge containing fyrite (shown).

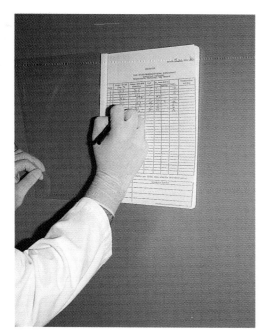

**3-29** The temperature, humidity, and atmosphere must be recorded daily.

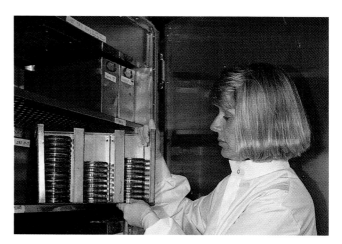

**3-30** Media should be incubated as soon as possible after inoculation. As shown here, inoculated media is arranged in an orderly manner to minimize errors and avoid contamination.

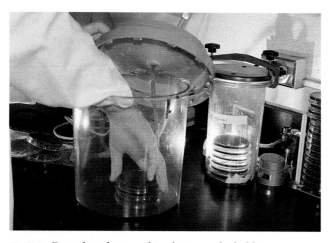

**3-31** Prereduced anaerobic plates can be held in an anaerobic holding jar for a short time before and after inoculation.

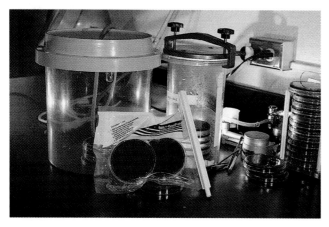

**3-32** An anaerobic atmosphere can also be created in an anaerobic pouch that holds only two plates or in an anaerobic jar for three or more plates.

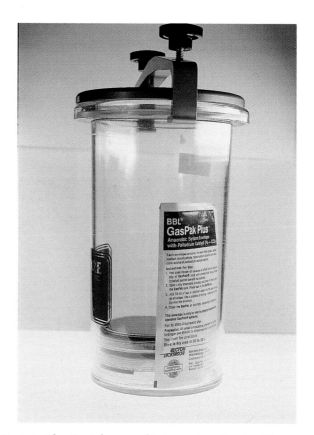

**3-33** The GasPak anaerobic jar system (Becton Dickinson Microbiology Systems, Cockeysville, Md.) contains a hydrogen and $CO_2$ generator envelope, a disposable methylene blue indicator, and a catalyst basket in the lid.

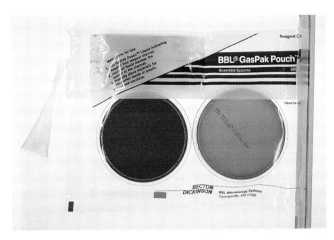

**3-34**   The GasPak anaerobic pouch (Becton Dickinson Microbiology Systems, Cockeysville, Md.) is based on the same principle. The bag is oxygen impermeable, and the system contains its own gas-generating kit and cold catalyst.

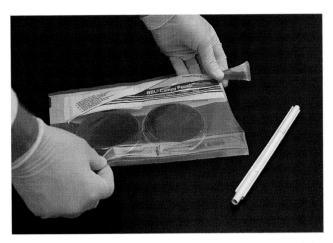

**3-35**   For recovery of *Campylobacter* spp., a microaerophilic atmosphere can also be created in a pouch or a jar.

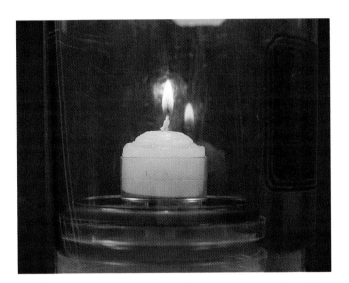

**3-36**   Recovery of some fastidious microorganisms (i.e., *Bordetella pertussis, Neisseria gonorrhoeae*) requires a microaerophilic atmosphere (decreased $O_2$) that can be created by burning a candle in a closed jar.

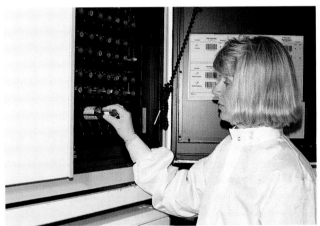

**3-37**   The technologist is placing a blood culture bottle into the BACTEC 9240 Fluorescent automated blood culture system (Becton Dickinson Diagnostic Instrument Systems, Sparks, Md.). Each bottle is entered into a cell of the incubator and monitored every 10 minutes by a photocell feedback system to a computer.

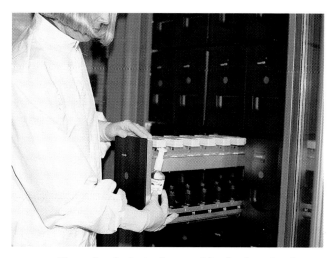

**3-38**  The technologist is placing a blood culture bottle into the ESP instrument (Difco Laboratories, Detroit, Mich.). A connector is placed onto the top of the bottle before incubation. Each bottle is entered into a cell of the incubator and monitored every 10 minutes by a pressure gauge interfaced to a computer.

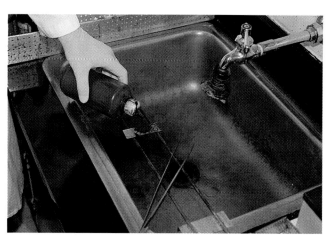

**3-39**  Direct smears should be methanol-fixed and stained as soon as possible after the slide is prepared and dried.

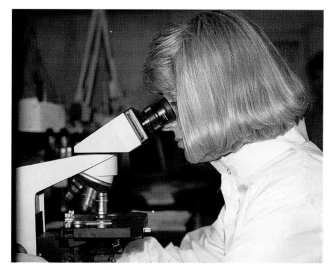

**3-40**  Stained smears should be read immediately after staining. Abnormal results must be telephoned immediately to a physician; the date and time of the call must be documented. The type of urgent results that require a verbal report should be listed in the procedure manual.

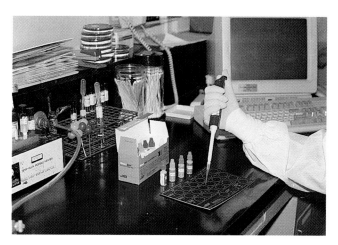

**3-41**  Specimen processing should also include a variety of rapid direct tests that can assist the physician with the patient's diagnosis. Examples include direct antigen tests, such as a cryptococcal antigen latex agglutination test shown here.

# CHAPTER 4 *Gram Stain*

The Gram stain is used to classify microorganisms on the basis of their Gram staining characteristics, size, shape, and arrangement of cells. It is one of the few tests in clinical microbiology that can assist in the rapid, presumptive diagnosis of an infectious disease. It is also used to assess the quality of the clinical specimen based on the somatic cellular content. Bacteria and fungi stain gram-positive, gram-negative, or gram-variable. The gram-variable appearance can be due to over- or under-decolorization, age of the microorganism, influence of antimicrobial treatment and other factors. The staining reaction is dependent on the microbial cell wall composition. The tightly cross-linked peptidoglycan layer and the teichoic acid found in gram-positive microorganisms cause them to be resistant to acetone-alcohol decolorization. They retain the crystal violet stain and are purple in color. The lipopolysaccharide-rich cell wall of gram-negative microorganisms is disrupted by acetone-alcohol and the crystal violet leaks out of the less tightly cross-linked cell wall structure. The safranin counter stain can then be seen, rendering gram-negative organisms pink in color.

The size of most bacteria ranges from a large cell (10µm to 30µm in length) to a small cell (1µm to 3µm in length). The shapes of bacteria are usually described as coccal, bacillary, or coccobacillary, and the arrangements as pairs, clusters, chains, branching, filamentous or coryneform. Yeast can be seen as single cells, often with budding and/or hyphal filaments. Microorganisms may be seen intracellularly within somatic cells. Staining characteristics of individual bacterial cells include bipolar, beaded and irregular. Ends may appear rounded, pointed, flattened, or swollen. Microorganisms other than bacteria and yeast observed in Gram stains, although they are better characterized with other stains, are *Trichomonas* trophozoites, *Pneumocystis carinii* cysts, *Toxoplasma gondii* trophozoites, and *Strongyloides* larvae.

Somatic cells can also be seen in a Gram stain, best observed with methanol-fixed smears as shown here. White blood cells (WBC) and epithelial cells tend to stain a pink color whereas red blood cells (RBC) appear tan to buff colored. The presence and rough quantitation of somatic cells should be noted when interpreting a Gram stain.

Gram stains should be examined under low power magnification (10× objective) for the quality of overall staining, the thickness, and for evaluation of somatic cells; microorganisms should be observed under oil immersion (100× objective).

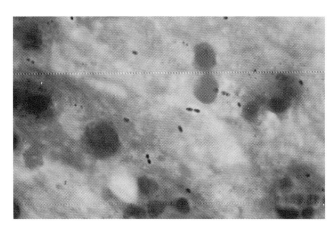

**4-1**  Polymorphonuclear leukocytes (PMN) and gram-positive lancet-shaped diplococci suggestive of *Streptococcus pneumoniae* (×1250). The clear area surrounding the bacterial cells is suggestive of a capsule. A rapid direct bacterial antigen test may be performed on the clinical specimen to confirm the organism identification.

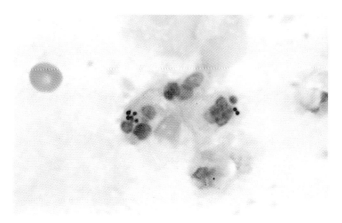

**4-2**  PMN, red blood cells (RBC), and gram-positive cocci in pairs.

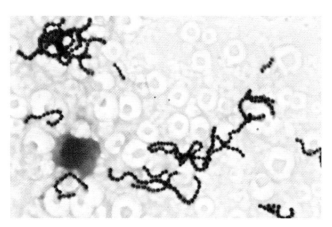

**4-3**  Gram-positive cocci in chains resembling streptococci (×1250).

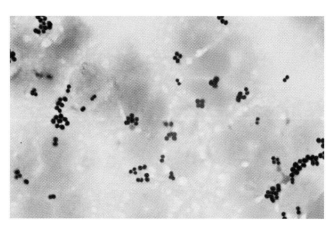

**4-4**  Gram-positive cocci in pairs, tetrads, and clusters resembling staphylococci (×1250).

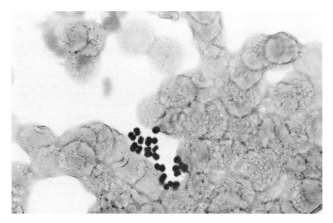

**4-5**  RBC and gram-positive cocci in tetrads (×1250). Cocci are somewhat large, irregular, and vary in size suggestive of coagulase-negative staphylococci, *Aerococcus*, or *Stomatococcus* spp. *Staphylococcus aureus* cells are uniform in size and appear as clusters of small cocci (~1 μm in diameter).

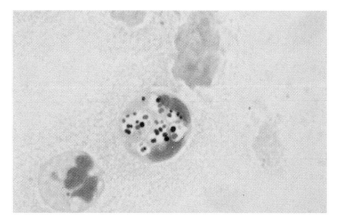

**4-6**  Intracellular, unevenly stained, pleomorphic, round, and gram-variable cocci (×1250). In such cases, the gram-variable appearance may be due to phagocytosis and partial degradation of the microorganisms by the PMN.

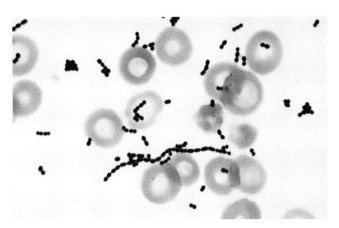

**4-7** RBC and gram-positive cocci in pairs, short and long chains, and clusters suggestive of mixed staphylococci and streptococci (×1250).

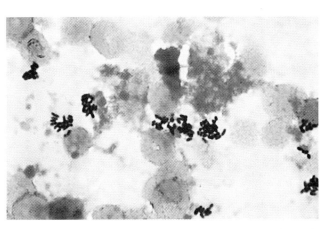

**4-8** RBC and small to medium gram-positive bacilli with palisading and angular arrangements (×1250). Some appear coccobacillary, diphtheroidlike, and pleomorphic, which is suggestive of corynebacteria or *Listeria monocytogenes*.

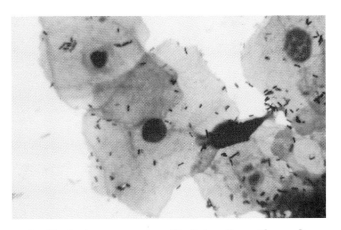

**4-9** Vaginal squamous epithelial cells with medium, straight gram-positive/gram-variable bacilli with rounded or blunt ends, some in chains, suggestive of lactobacilli (×1250). Clear background and sharp epithelial cell edges typical of pattern seen with normal vaginal secretions.

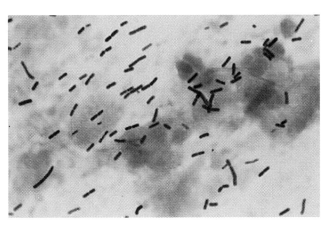

**4-10** Disintegrated WBC and pleomorphic large gram-positive bacilli resembling *Clostridium perfringens* or, rarely, *Bacillus* spp. (×1250).

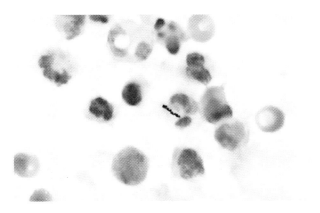

**4-11** PMN and large gram-positive bacilli (×1250). There appear to be two bacilli that are irregular in shape and staining, giving the appearance of cocci in chains. The beaded appearance may be due to the presence of spores, partial digestion by the PMN, or because the structure is a small piece of fungal hyphae, which stains unevenly with the Gram stain.

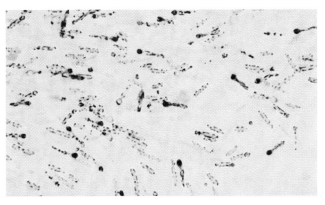

**4-12** Large. gram-variable bacilli with swollen ends (×1250). Some cells appear as drumsticks, suggestive of *Clostridium tetani*.

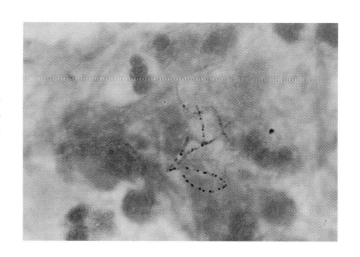

**4-13**    PMN and long, thin, beaded, branching, unevenly stained gram-positive filaments suggestive of *Actinomyces* or *Nocardia* spp. (×1250). The genus may be confirmed with a modified (partial) acid-fast stain. *Nocardia* spp. are partially acid-fast.

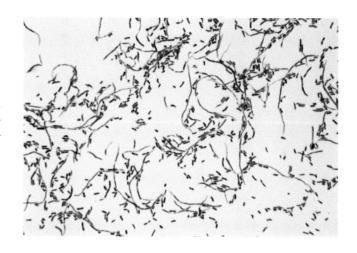

**4-14**    Branching, filamentous, slender gram-positive bacilli. If obtained from an aerobic colony, this morphology is suggestive of *Oerskovia* spp. (×1250). From a colony of a strict anaerobe, this morphology suggests *Clostridium* spp.

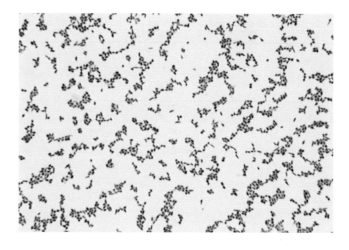

**4-15**    *Oerskovia* spp. fragment into coccoid forms after prolonged incubation (×1250).

# Gram-Negative Microorganisms

Gram-negative microorganisms can appear as cocci, coccobacilli, and bacilli. Cocci can appear as singles, in pairs with flattened adjacent sides, and in clusters. Coccobacilli are usually small to medium in size. Bacilli can vary in appearance from small, faintly staining rods to large, plump rods with bipolar staining.

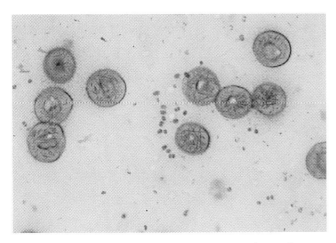

**4-16** RBC and gram-negative cocci in singles and pairs. The adjacent sides of the diplococci appear flattened (×1250). This microorganism is *Neisseria meningitidis* stained from a blood culture broth.

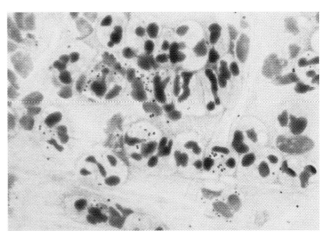

**4-17** Urethral discharge with PMN and intracellular gram-negative diplococci suggestive of *Neisseria gonorrhoeae* (×1250).

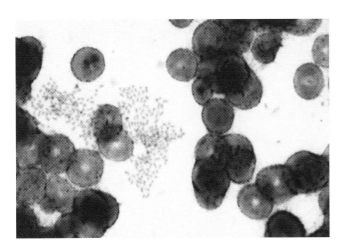

**4-18** RBC and small gram-negative coccobacilli in clusters (×1250). This microorganism, stained from the blood culture broth, was identified as *Brucella* spp.

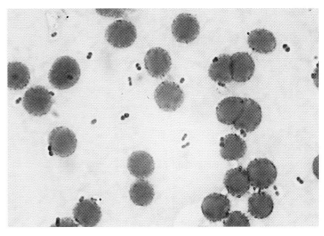

**4-19** RBC and gram-negative coccobacilli in pairs subsequently identified as *Acinetobacter* spp. in a blood culture broth (×1250). The morphology resembles *Neisseria* spp. and can be easily misinterpreted as gram-negative diplococci. The HACEK group of fastidious gram-negative bacilli (*Haemophilus*, *Actinobacillus*, *Cardiobacterium*, *Eikenella*, and *Kingella*), often detected as agents of endocarditis, can also appear as small coccobacilli.

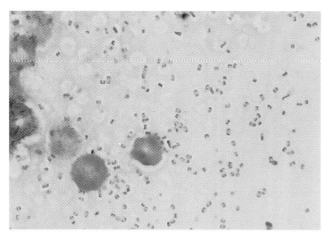

**4-20** RBC and plump gram-negative bacilli with bipolar staining in a blood culture broth, suggestive of "coliforms," belonging to the *Enterobacteriaceae* (×1250). The short, thick bacilli are characteristic of *Escherichia coli.*

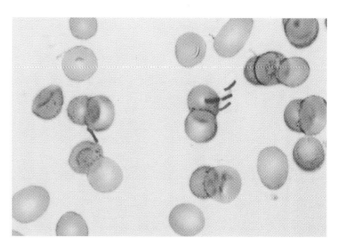

**4-21** RBC and long gram-negative bacilli with rounded ends suggestive of *Proteus* or *Pseudomonas* spp. (×1250) in a blood culture broth.

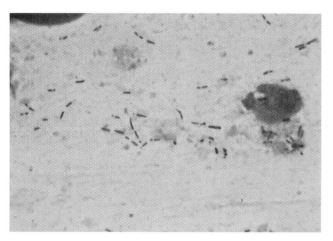

**4-22** Poorly differentiated PMN and slender pleomorphic gram-negative bacilli suggestive of *Haemophilus* spp. or anaerobes (×1250).

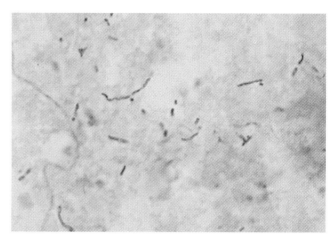

**4-23** Extremely pleomorphic, variably staining gram-negative bacilli with pointed ends suggestive of *Fusobacterium* spp. (×1250).

A

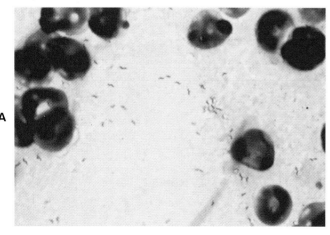

B

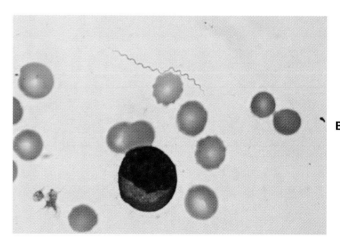

**4-24 A,** PMN, RBC, and slightly curved, comma-shaped, gull-wing, and S-shaped microorganisms suggest *Campylobacter* spp. (×1250). **B,** Wright's stain of *Borrelia* sp. seen in a peripheral blood smear (×1250). These helical bacteria measure approximately 0.3 μm in diameter and up to 15 μm in length with up to 10 loose coils.

# Yeast

Yeast cells are larger than bacteria, usually ranging from 8 to 15 μm in size. They can appear as single cells with buds, in clusters, and with hyphal filaments. Staining of cells can be somewhat speckled rather than confluent.

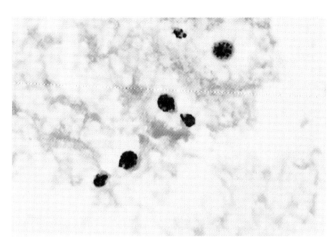

**4-25** Round budding yeast cells with single blastoconidia and speckled, uneven staining surrounded by clear halos (stain excluded by the polysaccharide capsule) suggestive of *Cryptococcus* spp. (×1250).

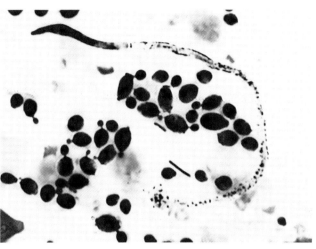

**4-26** Oval budding yeast cells and an irregularly stained pseudohyphal filament suggestive of *Candida* spp. (×1250).

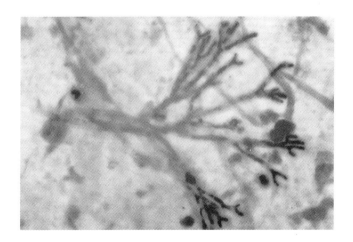

**4-27** Unevenly stained 3 to 4 μm width nondematiaceous hyphae with parallel walls and 45° branching and septations suggestive of *Aspergillus* spp. (×1250).

# CHAPTER 5 *Micrococcaceae*

Three genera of the family *Micrococcaceae* have been associated with infections in humans: *Staphylococcus, Micrococcus,* and *Stomatococcus.* Of these, *Staphylococcus* spp. are by far the most common cause of human infections. Both *Micrococcus* and *Stomatococcus* spp. can be found in the environment, as normal flora of the skin and respiratory tract, and as pathogens associated with catheter tips and other hardware.

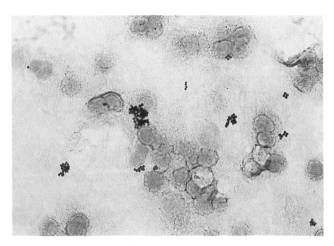

**5-1 Gram stain** showing RBCs and gram-positive cocci in pairs, tetrads, and grapelike clusters suggestive of *Micrococcaceae* (×1250). In this figure, the microorganisms are staphylococci.

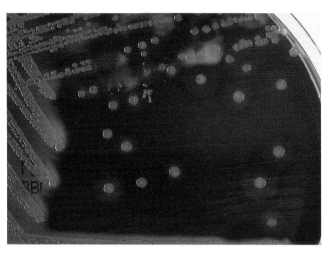

**5-2 Colonies of *Staphylococcus aureus* on 5% sheep blood agar.** Typical appearance of *S. aureus* colonies is creamy/buff colored colonies surrounded by a zone of complete β hemolysis.

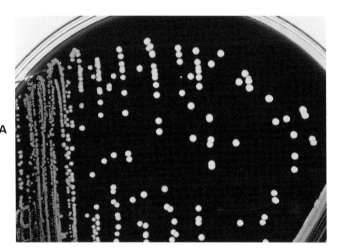
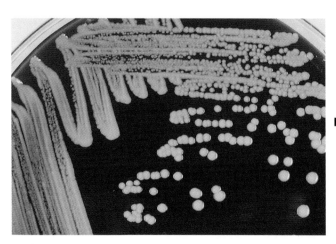

**5-3 A, Colonies of coagulase-negative staphylococci on 5% sheep blood agar.** Typical colonies of coagulase-negative staphylococci are nonhemolytic and white. **B, Colonies of *Micrococcus* spp. on 5% sheep blood agar.** Typical colonies of *Micrococcus* appear lemon-yellow. *Micrococcus* spp. usually grow more slowly than staphylococci, sometimes requiring 48 hours of incubation before colonies are visible.

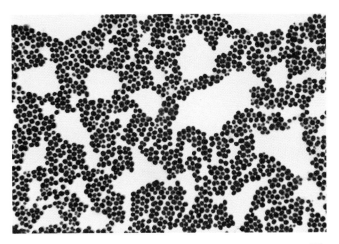

**5-4  Gram stain of *Micrococcus* species.** Microscopically, micrococci are larger than staphylococci and appear in tetrads rather than grapelike clusters (×1250).

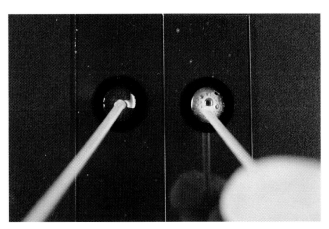

**5-5  Catalase test.** The test is performed by adding 3% hydrogen peroxide ($H_2O_2$) to a colony on a glass slide or by adding colony paste on a wooden stick to a drop of $H_2O_2$ on a slide, as shown here. The appearance of bubbles indicates that the enzyme, catalase, has hydrolyzed $H_2O_2$ into oxygen plus water. Staphylococci and micrococci are differentiated from other aerobic gram-positive cocci by a positive catalase test (*right*). No bubbles appear in a negative test result (*left*).

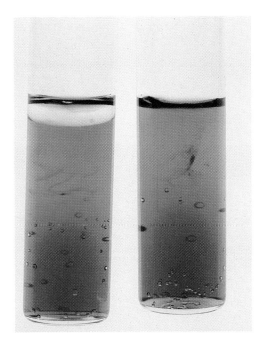

**5-6  Fermentation of glucose** is one of the methods used to differentiate *Staphylococcus* spp. from *Micrococcus* spp. When grown in an oxidation-fermentation (OF) medium, staphylococci produce acid (*yellow color*) from glucose under anaerobic conditions, created by layering mineral oil over the surface of the agar (*tube on the left*). The microorganism also utilizes glucose aerobically (*tube on the right*).

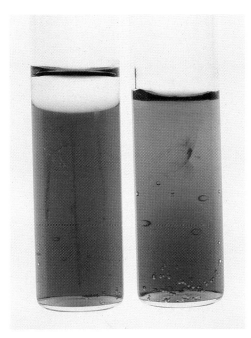

**5-7  Glucose oxidation in OF medium.** *Micrococcus* spp. oxidize glucose (*right, yellow color in the open tube*), but do not ferment the carbohydrate (*left, no color change [green] in the overlaid tube*). The acid reaction produced by oxidative organisms appears at the surface and gradually extends throughout the medium.

**5-8   Bacitracin susceptibility test.** Susceptibility to 0.04 units of the antibiotic bacitracin is also used to differentiate *Staphylococcus* spp. from *Micrococcus* spp. The surface of a Mueller-Hinton agar plate is inoculated with the microorganism, the disk is applied, and the plate is incubated overnight. Staphylococci are resistant to 0.04 units bacitracin (*zone of inhibition less than or equal to 9 mm, organism on the right*) and micrococci are susceptible (*zones of inhibition greater than or equal to 10 mm, organism on the left*).

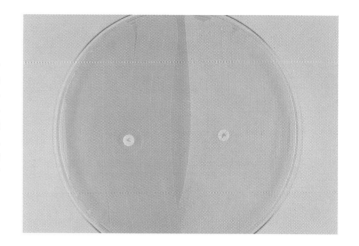

**5-9   Slide coagulase test performed on a glass slide.** Cells from a fresh colony are inoculated into saline to make a smooth suspension (*left*), and a drop of rabbit plasma is added. If the organism possesses bound coagulase ("clumping factor"), the enzyme acts on fibrinogen in the plasma and causes clumping of the bacteria, as shown on the right. *S. aureus* is the most common pathogen among the catalase-positive, gram-positive cocci, and it is easily differentiated from other staphylococci by the coagulase test. Coagulase is a thermostable enzyme found primarily in *S. aureus*. There are two forms of coagulase: bound and free.

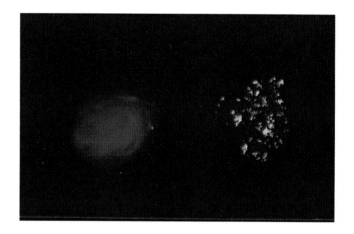

**5-10   The tube coagulase test** detects free coagulase. Microorganisms are incubated in plasma for 2 to 4 hours, and the tubes are turned on their sides, as shown here. Free coagulase acts on prothrombin and fibrinogen in rabbit plasma and forms a fibrin clot (*tube on the left*).

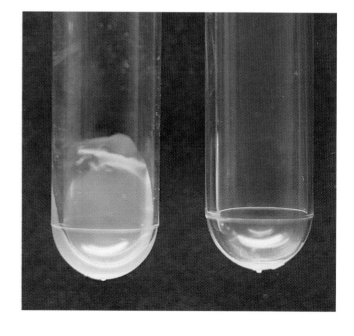

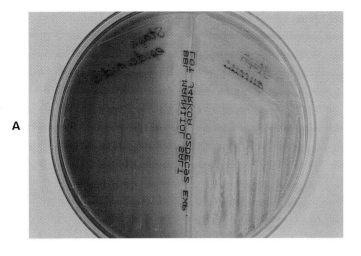

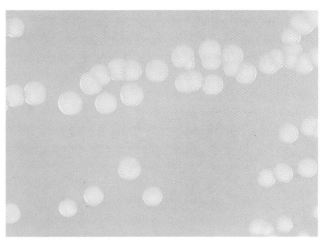

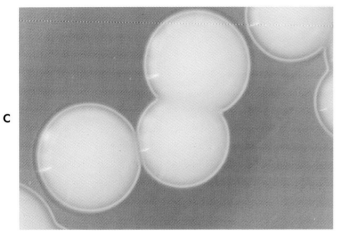

**5-11  Mannitol salt agar. A,** Mannitol salt agar differentiates *S. aureus* from other catalase-positive gram-positive cocci. The medium contains 7.5% NaCl, which inhibits the growth of many microorganisms. *S. aureus* will grow and ferment mannitol resulting in acid production, which causes the phenol red indicator to change from pink to yellow (*growth on right half of this plate*). The left half of the agar plate was inoculated with coagulase-negative staphylococci. Coagulase-negative staphylococci will grow on the medium, but because the organism does not ferment mannitol, the phenol red indicator does not change in color, and the colonies and surrounding medium appear pink. **B,** Colonies of *Staphylococcus aureus* on mannitol salt agar (close-up). Medium surrounding colonies has turned yellow. **C,** Opaque, shiny, yellow colonies of *Staphylococcus aureus* on mannitol salt agar (close-up).

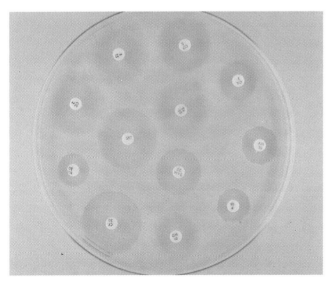

**5-12  Antimicrobial susceptibility testing of *S. aureus.*** Most community-acquired strains of *S. aureus* are resistant to penicillin.

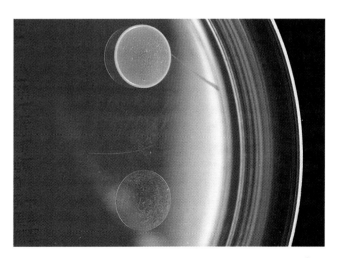

**5-13  Oxacillin screen plate.** Screening agar plate containing 6 μg/ml oxacillin in 4% NaCl-supplemented Mueller Hinton agar, used to detect methicillin (and oxacillin)-resistant *S. aureus* (MRSA). Oxacillin is used because it is a better indicator antibiotic. Growth that occurred after 24-hour incubation at 35°C from a spot of an inoculum of MRSA is shown on the top and the lack of growth of a methicillin-susceptible *S. aureus* on the bottom.

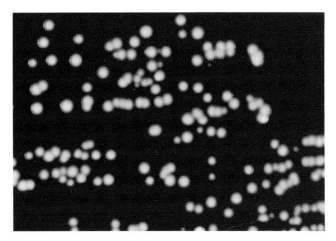

**5-14  Colonial morphology of *Staphylococcus saprophyticus* on 5% sheep blood agar.**
Colonies resemble those of coagulase-negative staphylococci.

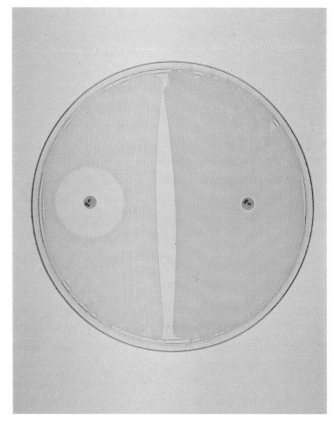

**5-15  Novobiocin susceptibility test,** used to differentiate *S. saprophyticus* (*resistant; microorganism on the right*) from other species of coagulase-negative staphylococci (*susceptible; microorganism on the left*) encountered in urine specimens.

# CHAPTER 6 *Streptococcaceae*

T he family *Streptococcaceae* and related genera include nine genera encountered in the clinical laboratory: *Aerococcus, Aloiococcus, Enterococcus, Gemella, Globicatella, Lactococcus, Leuconostoc, Pediococcus,* and *Streptococcus.* The more commonly isolated genera are illustrated here. The streptococci are catalase-negative, gram-positive, coccoid to coccobacillary in morphology, forming pairs and chains. Colonial morphology and hemolysis on 5% sheep blood agar are very helpful characteristics used for preliminary identification. Hemolysis is classified as alpha, beta, or gamma.

**6-1 Alpha hemolysis on 5% sheep blood agar plate.** Alpha hemolysis is an indistinct zone of partial lysis of red blood cells (RBC) causing a green to greenish-brown discoloration of the medium immediately surrounding the colony. Viridans streptococcal colonies and pneumococcal colonies are alphahemolytic.

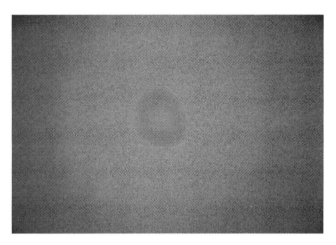

**6-2 Colony of alpha-hemolytic streptococci (×10).** Microscopic view of alpha-hemolysis showing the partially hemolyzed RBC immediately surrounding the colony.

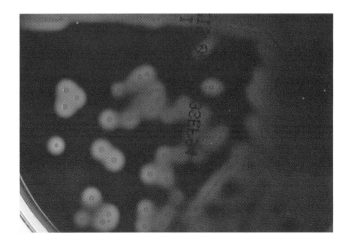

**6-3 Beta hemolysis on 5% sheep blood agar plate.** With beta hemolysis, there is complete lysis of RBC surrounding the colony that can readily be seen macroscopically.

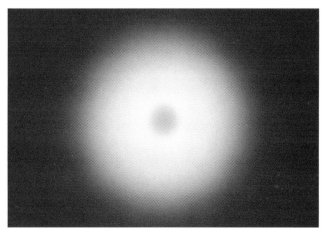

**6-4 Colony of beta-hemolytic streptococci (×10).** Microscopic view of beta hemolysis showing the clear, colorless zone around the streptococcal colonies in which the RBC have undergone complete destruction.

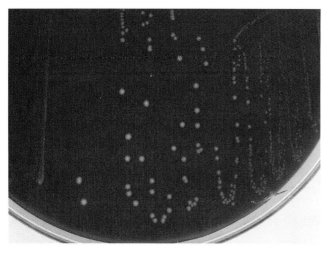

**6-5  Gamma hemolysis on 5% sheep blood agar.** *Gamma* is a term used to denote lack of hemolysis; the RBC surrounding the colonies are intact.

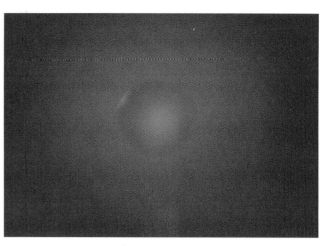

**6-6  Colony of nonhemolytic streptococci (×10).** Macroscopically, there is no apparent hemolytic activity or discoloration produced by the colony.

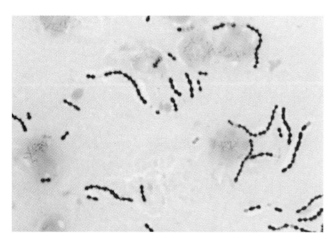

**6-7  Gram stain of streptococci in broth culture (×1250).** Gram stain of a positive blood culture broth demonstrating gram-positive cocci arranged in chains. Streptococci are normal microbiota in the upper respiratory tract and the gastrointestinal tract. For this reason, Gram stains of specimens from these sites are not helpful in diagnosing infections caused by the pathogenic streptococci, such as *S. pyogenes* and *S. pneumoniae*.

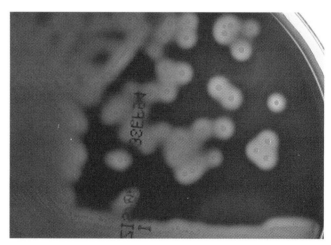

**6-8  Colonies of group A streptococci on 5% sheep blood agar.** Colonies of group A streptococci on 5% sheep blood agar are small and surrounded by wide zones of beta hemolysis.

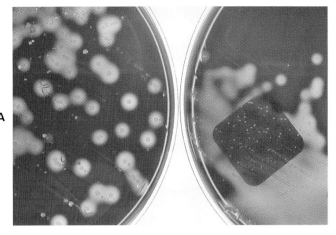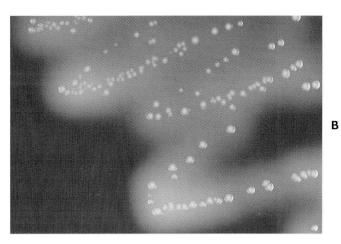

**6-9  A, Colonies of group A streptococci on 5% sheep blood agar (*left*) and Streptococcus selective agar (SSA) (*right*),** a primary selective isolation medium for group A streptococci. Observe that the colonies on the SSA are smaller as can be seen on the plate on the right. Groups C, F, and G can also be isolated from the upper respiratory tract, and their colonies can be confused with group A streptococci if 5% sheep blood agar is used. Inoculation of a selective medium such as this, containing sulfamethoxazole (23.75 µg/ml) and trimethoprim (1.25 µg/ml), inhibits the growth of nongroup A betahemolytic streptococci as well as staphylococci, viridans streptococci, and gram-negative bacilli. **B, Colonies of *Streptococcus pyogenes* on 5% sheep blood agar.** Colonies are small (1 mm), translucent, and surrounded by a wide zone of beta hemolysis.

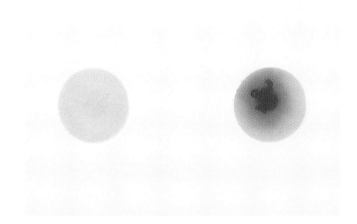

**6-10  PYR test.** The presence of an aminopeptidase enzyme that degrades the substrate PYR (L-pyrrolidonyl-β-naphthylamide) is a 10-minute presumptive test for group A streptococci (beta-hemolytic) and *Aerococcus, Enterococcus,* and *Gemella* (alpha- or nonhemolytic). A positive test is indicated by a red color (*disk on the right*).

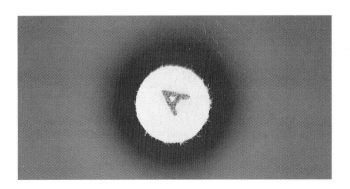

**6-11  Bacitracin susceptibility test.** The bacitracin susceptibility test is an alternative to the PYR test for the presumptive identification of group A beta-hemolytic streptococci. A 0.04-U bacitracin disk is placed on an inoculum of the microorganism on sheep blood agar. After overnight incubation at 35°C, any zone of inhibition is interpreted as a positive test, and the microorganism is presumptively identified as group A streptococci by bacitracin.

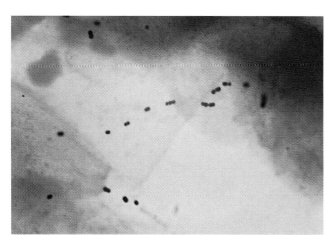

**6-12 Gram stain of vaginal secretions** showing epithelial cells and gram-positive cocci in pairs, suggestive of streptococci (×1250). Group B streptococci, *S. agalactiae*, can colonize the genitourinary tract of women, occasionally colonizing and infecting the neonate at delivery and therefore is the major cause of neonatal sepsis and meningitis. Microscopically, this species usually occurs in pairs, as shown in this figure.

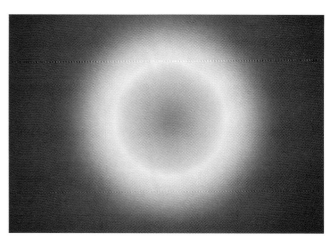

**6-13 Colonies of group B streptococci on 5% sheep blood agar (×10).** Group B streptococcal colonies are larger than other beta-hemolytic streptococci, but the hemolytic zone surrounding the colony is smaller; compare zone size of beta hemolysis with Figure 6-8 on p. 38.

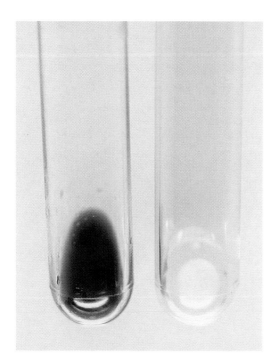

**6-14 Hippurate hydrolysis test.** Group B streptococci and some enterococci can hydrolyze sodium hippurate, resulting in the formation of glycine and sodium benzoate. A suspension of the microorganism is incubated for 2 hours at 35°C in a hippurate solution and then the indicator, ninhydrin, is added. Deamination of glycine, if it is present, is detected by the development of a purple color within 10 minutes (*tube on the left*). A negative reaction (*tube on the right*) remains colorless.

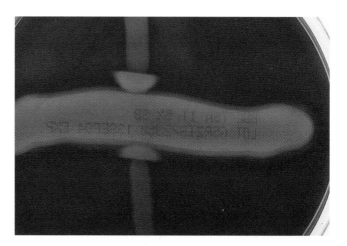

**6-15 CAMP Test.** A positive CAMP test for group B streptococci demonstrating the arrowhead-shaped enhancement of beta hemolysis that occurs when the hemolytic beta-toxin produced by *S. aureus* (the microorganism streaked horizontally across the sheep blood agar plate in this photograph) acts synergistically with the CAMP factor protein produced by Group B streptococci (streaked perpendicular to the staphylococcus but not quite touching). The CAMP test, which is named for its discoverers, Christie, Atkins, and Munch-Peterson, is an alternative to hippurate hydrolysis.

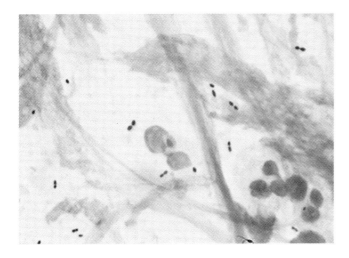

**6-16 Gram stain of respiratory secretions** demonstrating gram-positive, lancet-shaped diplococci suggestive of *Streptococcus pneumoniae.*

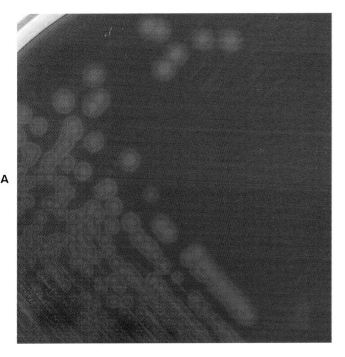

A

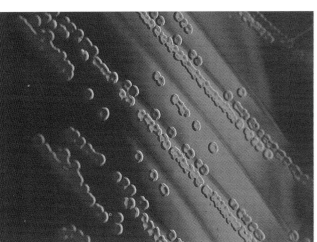

B

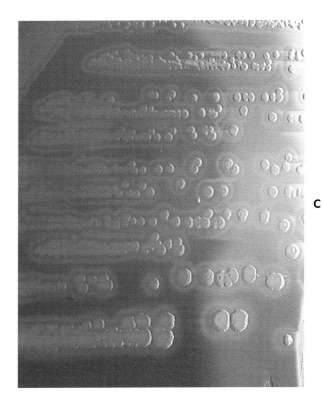

C

**6-17 A, Colonies of *Streptococcus pneumoniae* on 5% sheep blood agar.** These young colonies are round with complete edges, somewhat mucoid, and about 1 mm in diameter. They are surrounded by a zone of alpha hemolysis. **B, Colonies of *Streptococcus pneumoniae* on 5% sheep blood agar.** These slightly older colonies display the central indentation caused by the easily induced autolysis typical of *S. pneumoniae.* **C, Colonies of *Streptococcus pneumoniae* on 5% sheep blood agar.** Occasionally, *S. pneumoniae* colonies may simply flatten out as they age.

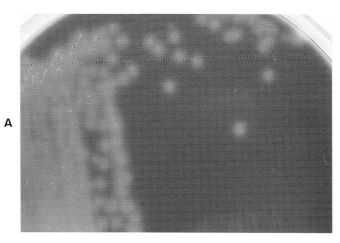
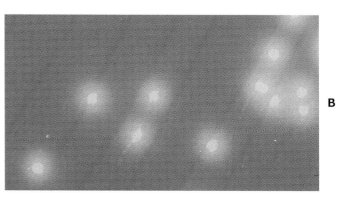

**6-18   A, Colonies of *Streptococcus pneumoniae* on chocolate agar.** Medium was incubated in $CO_2$, resulting in fairly large zones of alpha hemolysis. **B, Colonies of Streptococcus pneumoniae on chocolate agar (close-up).** Colonies are quite flat on chocolate agar.

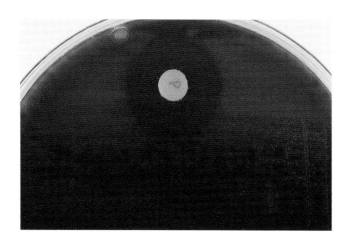

**6-19   Optochin susceptibility test.** Colonies of *Streptococcus pneumoniae* are inhibited by the antimicrobic optochin (ethylhydrocupreine hydrochloride) contained in the paper disk applied to the surface of an inoculated 5% sheep blood agar plate. A zone of greater than or equal to 14 mm in diameter is presumptive identification for *Streptococcus pneumoniae.* No zone of inhibition is consistent with viridans streptococci. Zones of less than 14 mm in diameter are questionable and should be confirmed with the bile solubility test.

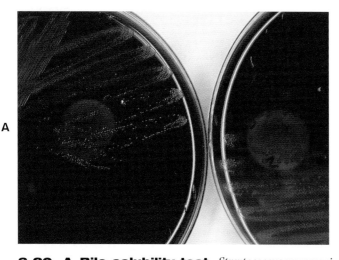
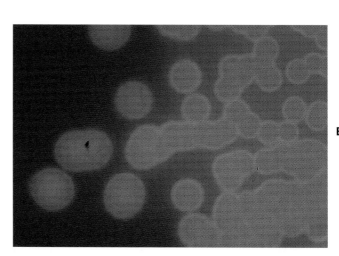

**6-20   A, Bile solubility test.** *Streptococcus pneumoniae* colonies will dissolve or lyse within 30 minutes at 35°C in the presence of 2% sodium desoxycholate. A drop of the reagent is applied directly to the colonies, which dissolve (*plate on the right*) if the organism is *Streptococcus pneumoniae.* Colonies on the blood agar plate on the left, also overlayed with bile, remain intact, indicating that the isolate is not *Streptococcus pneumoniae.* **B, Bile solubility test (*close-up*).** *Streptococcus pneumoniae* colonies have dissolved in the bile added to the plate surface. After the bile has evaporated, only the zone of hemolysis remains, as shown here.

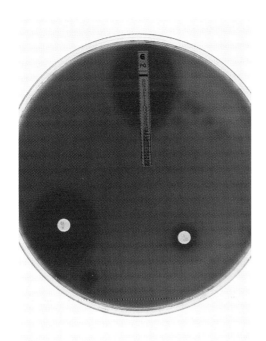

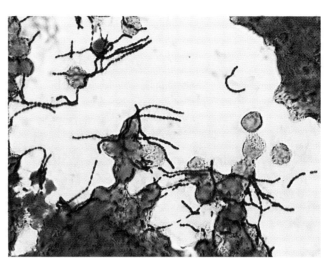

**6-22 Gram stain of a viridans streptococcus species in blood culture broth (×1250).** There are numerous species of the viridans streptococci group, which are normal mucosal microbiota in mammals. Only a few require identification to the species level, such as *S. bovis*. Microscopically, they usually appear in long chains, especially when recovered from a blood culture broth medium.

**6-21 Antimicrobial susceptibility testing of *Streptococcus pneumoniae*.** *Streptococcus pneumoniae* can be tested for penicillin resistance using a 10 unit penicillin disk, a 1 μg oxacillin disk or quantitatively with the E-test (AB Biodisk, Solna, Sweden), consisting of a plastic strip impregnated with increasing concentrations of the antibiotic (in this case, penicillin). Following overnight incubation, the point at which the elliptical zone of inhibition of growth of the isolate intersects the quantitative scale on the strip is interpreted as the minimal inhibitory concentration (MIC).

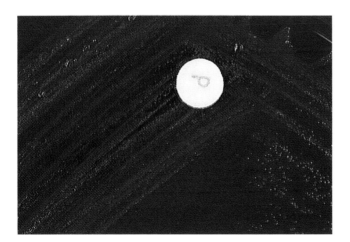

**6-23 Optochin susceptibility test** performed on a species of viridans streptococci. Colonies of viridans streptococci are resistant to optochin, distinguishing these commonly encountered organisms from *Streptococcus pneumoniae* (shown in Figure 6-19).

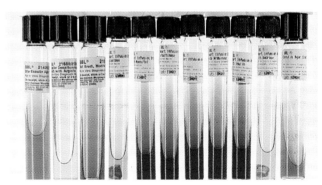

**6-24 Identification of viridans streptococci with conventional biochemical reactions.** Definitive identification requires several substrates including bile esculin, arginine decarboxylase, 6.5% NaCl, lactose, mannitol, raffinose, sorbitol, arabinose, inulin, sucrose, and esculin (*shown here*). Other characteristics such as urease, Voges-Proskauer reaction, bile insolubility, optochin resistance, and failure to grow at 10°C and 45°C, will help to identify the clinically significant isolates.

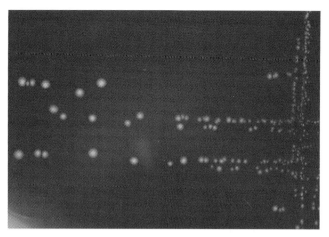

**6-25 Colonies of *Pediococcus* spp. on 5% sheep blood agar.** *Pediococcus* spp. resemble viridans streptococci in their colonial morphology, but microscopically they appear as pairs, tetrads, and clusters. They may be distinguished from other alpha-hemolytic microorganisms by their resistance to vancomycin (30 μg disk) (see Figure 6-26) and growth in 6.5% NaCl broth. They are also bile esculin-positive, but PYR-negative.

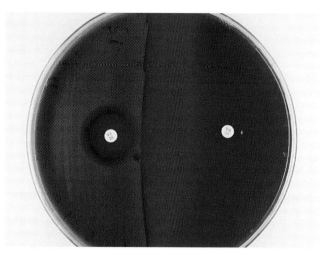

**6-26 Vancomycin susceptibility test.** *Pediococcus* spp. are distinguished from other alpha-hemolytic organisms by their resistance to vancomycin. There is no zone of inhibition surrounding the vancomycin disk placed on an inoculum of *Pediococcus* spp. (*right side of plate*) compared to a zone of inhibition surrounding the viridans streptococcus (*left side of plate*).

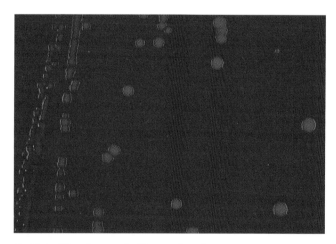

**6-27 Nonhemolytic colonies on 5% sheep blood agar plate.** In the family *Streptococcaceae*, the nonhemolytic organisms include the *Enterococcus* spp., some strains of viridans streptococci, *Lactococcus* spp., and *Leuconostoc* spp.

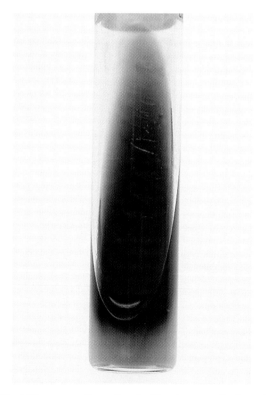

**6-28 Bile esculin slant.** *Streptococcus bovis* and the enterococci can grow in the presence of 40% bile and can hydrolyze esculin to esculetin. Esculetin and ferric citrate form a black complex in the agar, which contains 40% oxgall. A negative slant remains tan colored (no color change) compared to black colored slant (positive shown here).

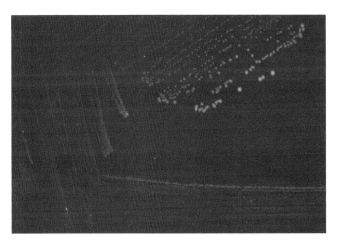

**6-29 Colonies of *Enterococcus* spp. on 5% sheep blood agar plate.** The colonies are raised, white to gray-white, range from 0.5 to 1.5 mm in size, and are usually nonhemolytic.

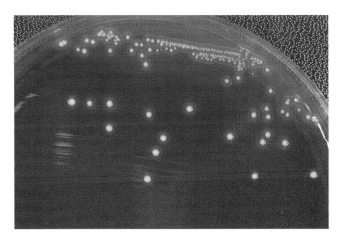

**6-31 Colonies of *Leuconostoc* spp. on 5% sheep blood agar plate.** Initially the colonies resemble *Enterococcus* spp. as described in Figure 6-29. Upon continued incubation (48 to 72 hours), a weak alpha hemolysis develops. Generally, these microorganisms can be distinguished from *Enterococcus* spp. by their resistance to vancomycin and by gas formation from glucose in Lactobacilli MRS broth (Difco Laboratories, Detroit, Mich.).

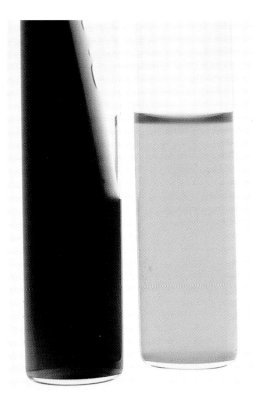

**6-30 Bile esculin slant and 6.5% NaCl broth.** The bile esculin slant (*left*) is black (positive), indicating that the microorganism can grow in the presence of bile and hydrolyze esculin. Growth in a broth containing a salt concentration of 6.5% (*tube on right*) is indicated by turbidity and a change in the indicator from pink to yellow following overnight incubation. The reactions shown here confirm the identification of *Enterococcus* spp. A positive PYR test (Figure 6-10) may also be used to confirm the identification of suspected *Enterococcus* spp. Nonenterococcal group D streptococci (*S. bovis*) are unable to grow in the presence of 6.5% NaCl broth.

# CHAPTER 7 *Aerobic Gram-Positive Bacilli and Actinomyces spp.*

C ommon genera of aerobic gram-positive bacilli include *Bacillus, Corynebacterium, Erysipelothrix, Gardnerella* (gram-variable), *Lactobacillus,* and *Listeria.* Rare clinical isolates include species of *Arcanobacterium, Oerskovia,* and *Rhodococcus.* Also included in this section are *Nocardia* and *Streptomyces,* genera containing filamentous, branching, gram-positive bacilli.

Preliminary differentiation among these genera is based on microscopic morphology and the catalase reaction. *Bacillus* spp., *Corynebacterium* spp., *Listeria, Oerskovia,* and *Rhodococcus* spp. are catalase-positive. Of these, *Bacillus* spp. is the only spore former. More examples of the microscopic morphologies of the gram-positive bacilli are presented in the Gram stain section.

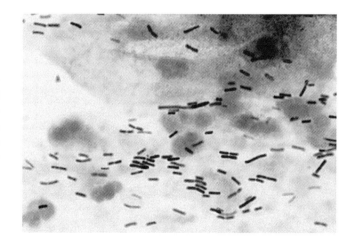

**7-1 Gram stain of *Bacillus* spp.** Large, gram-positive bacilli with squared-off ends measuring 0.8 × 7.5 μm, occurring singly and in chains (×1250). They may appear gram-variable. Some species demonstrate endospores, which may be located centrally or terminally along the bacilli. The microscopic morphology may resemble that of *Clostridium* spp.

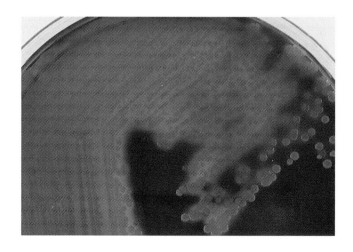

**7-2 Colonies of *Bacillus* spp. on 5% sheep blood agar.** Colonies of *Bacillus subtilis* are smooth, round, and surrounded by a zone of beta hemolysis. Colonies can also appear rough and dry with shaggy edges.

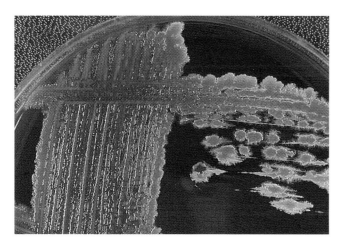

**7-3 Colonies of *Bacillus* spp. on 5% sheep blood agar.** Some species of *Bacillus* are nonhemolytic with mucoid and spreading colonies resembling the *Enterobacteriaceae* and *Pseudomonas* spp. Colonies of *Bacillus anthracis,* the major human pathogen, are usually nonhemolytic. This figure shows an environmental *Bacillus* sp. that rarely causes human infections.

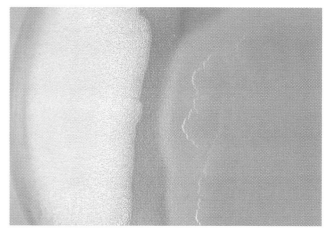

**7-4 Growth of *Bacillus* spp. on egg yolk agar.** Reaction on egg yolk agar is one of the characteristics used to identify *Bacillus* spp. *Bacillus cereus* is one of many species that produce the enzyme lecithinase, demonstrated by a zone of opacity (whitish color in the agar) extending away from the bacterial growth, as shown on the left. Lipase activity can also be detected on egg yolk agar, demonstrated by an oily looking sheen on the surface of the bacterial growth but not extending onto the agar, as shown on the right.

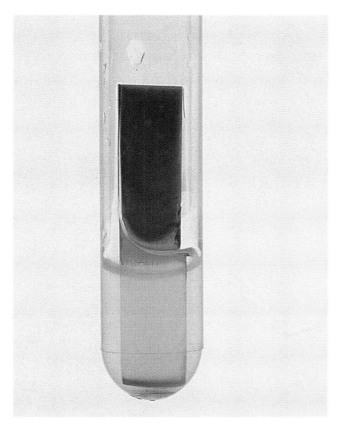

**7-5 Gelatin hydrolysis test.** Many *Bacillus* spp. secrete proteolytic enzymes that can hydrolyze gelatin. In the method shown in this figure, exposed, undeveloped x-ray film is used as the substrate for detection of gelatinase activity. Hydrolysis destroys the film's gelatin coating, leaving only the clear photographic film where the strip was immersed in the organism suspension.

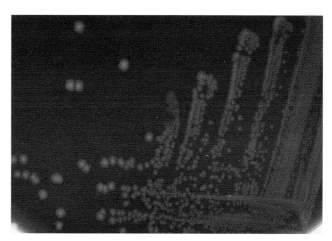

**7-6 Colonies of *Listeria monocytogenes* on 5% sheep blood agar.** Colonies of *Listeria monocytogenes* are small (less than 1 mm in diameter), smooth, irregular, and translucent. The colonies are surrounded by a very characteristic narrow zone of beta hemolysis on 5% sheep blood agar and may be confused with group B beta-hemolytic streptococci. Differentiating characteristics include *Listeria's* narrow zone of beta hemolysis, positive catalase production, and growth on bile and hydrolysis of esculin. Both species hydrolyze hippurate.

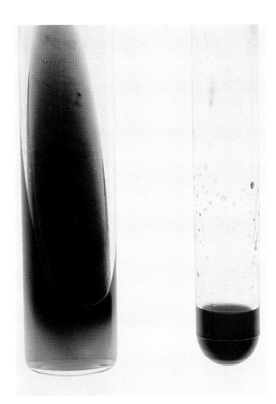

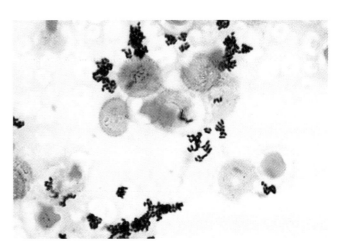

**7-8 Gram stain of *Corynebacterium* spp. (×1250).** Small gram-positive bacilli appearing in palisades, V, and L forms resembling Chinese letters. Most of the *Corynebacterium* spp. isolated in the clinical laboratory are normal flora of the skin and mucous membranes. It is difficult to differentiate the nonpathogenic species from the pathogenic, *C. diphtheriae* and *C. jeikeium*, on the basis of the Gram stain.

**7-7 Esculin hydrolysis test.** Most strains of *Listeria monocytogenes* can hydrolyze esculin in less than 2 hours. This photograph shows positive reactions for bile esculin (*tube on left*) and hippurate (*right*). These tests are described in Figure 6-14 on p. 40 and Figure 6-28 on p. 44.

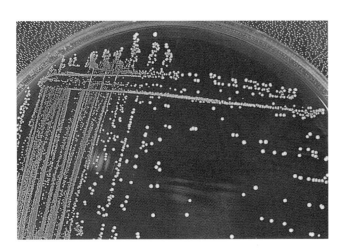

**7-9 Colonies of *C. jeikeium* on 5% sheep blood agar.** Colonies are smooth and whitish following overnight incubation in 5% to 10% $CO_2$. This species can cause life-threatening sepsis.

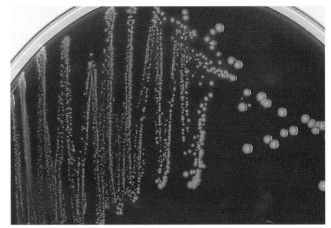

**7-10 Colonies of *C. diphtheriae* on 5% sheep blood agar.** *Corynebacterium diphtheriae* grow well on 5% sheep blood agar as whitish, opaque colonies.

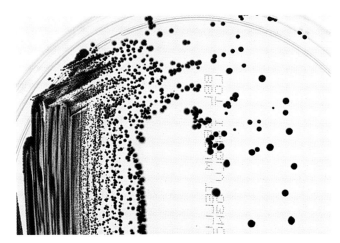

**7-11 Colonies of *C. diphtheriae* on Tinsdale agar.** A selective medium should be used along with sheep blood agar whenever *Corynebacterium diphtheriae* is suspected, as well as to differentiate *C. diphtheriae* from other corynebacteria. On the selective medium cystine tellurite agar or potassium tellurite (Tinsdale) agar, the colonies of *Corynebacterium diphtheriae* have a gunmetal, gray-black appearance.

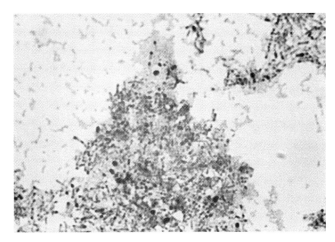

**7-12 Loeffler methylene blue stain.** *C. diphtheriae* demonstrate metachromatic granules when stained with either Loeffler methylene blue stain or Neisser stain. The stain is best performed on colonies grown on a Loeffler agar slant. Metachromatic deposits are reddish purple in Loeffler methylene blue stain.

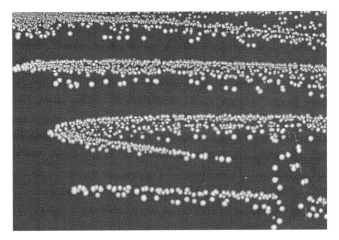

**7-13 Colonies of *Corynebacterium* spp.** Some *Corynebacterium* spp. (often called diphtheroids) appear as nonhemolytic, gray-white, small colonies and can easily be confused with colonies of streptococci, especially when isolated from the respiratory tract. Some species appear white and opaque resembling coagulase-negative staphylococci.

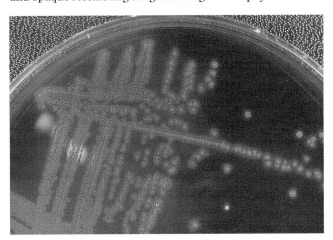

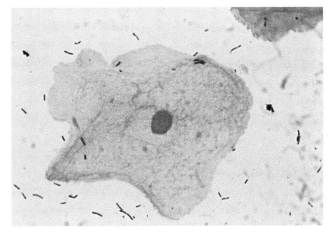

**7-14 Gram stain of *Lactobacillus* spp. in vaginal secretions.** *Lactobacillus* spp. appear as long, non-spore-forming gram-positive bacilli. They may also appear as short and pleomorphic coccobacilli. When they appear microscopically as coccobacilli, they can be misidentified as streptococci. Lactobacilli are normal flora of the upper respiratory tract, intestinal tract, and vagina, although they often fail to grow in culture.

**7-15 Colonies of *Lactobacillus* spp.** Colonies are alpha-hemolytic resembling viridans streptococci and *Erysipelothrix*. It may be necessary to differentiate these genera depending on the specimen source. In most cases, both lactobacilli and streptococci are normal flora and do not require identification. They are usually resistant to vancomycin. Growth on TSI agar will differentiate *Erysipelothrix* from lactobacilli, which are unable to grow.

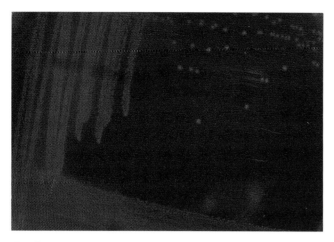

**7-16 Colonies of *Erysipelothrix rhusiopathiae*.**
Colonies are smooth, small (less than 1.0 mm in diameter), and transparent. A greenish color and/or α/hemolysis appears as the colonies age.

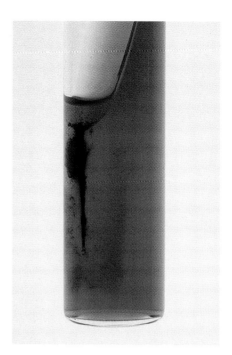

**7-17 *Erysipelothrix rhusiopathiae* on triple sugar iron (TSI) agar.** *Erysipelothrix rhusiopathiae* demonstrates H₂S production along the stab line in a TSI agar slant within 48 hours of incubation at 35°C. This is a helpful feature that separates this organism from other gram-positive bacilli.

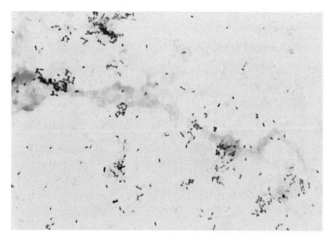

**7-18 Gram stain of *Gardnerella vaginalis* (×1250).** *Gardnerella vaginalis* is a small, gram-positive to gram-variable rod-like microorganism that can be isolated from the genitourinary tract of humans. This organism was at one time included in the genera *Corynebacterium* and *Haemophilus*.

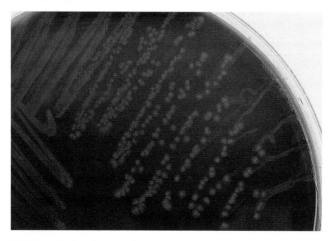

**7-19 Colonies of *Gardnerella vaginalis* on chocolate agar.** After 24 hours of incubation, colonies of *Gardnerella vaginalis* appear as tiny, pinpoint colonies on chocolate agar. Isolation of the microorganism is nonspecific for the diagnosis of bacterial vaginosis, since as many as 50% of women are colonized asymptomatically with *G. vaginalis*.

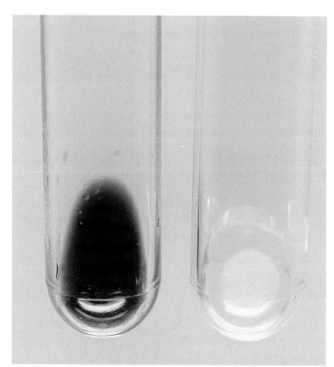

**7-20 Hippurate hydrolysis test.** *G. vaginalis* hydrolyzes sodium hippurate. This microorganism hydrolyzes 1% aqueous sodium hippurate following a 2-hour incubation at 35°C as described in Figure 6-14 on p. 40. A positive reaction is the development of a purple color within 10 minutes after the addition of ninhydrin. A negative reaction is colorless.

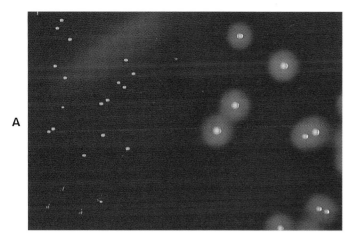

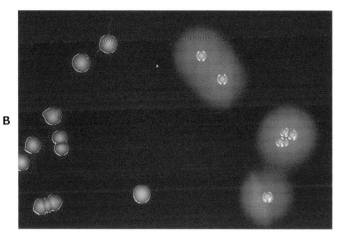

**7-21 A, Colonies of** *Arcanobacterium* *haemolyticum* **(left) and** *Streptococcus pyo-* *genes* **(right).** Colonies of *Arcanobacterium haemolyticum* are tiny (0.1 to 0.5 mm in diameter), beta-hemolytic after 48 hours, and can be confused with streptococci when isolated from a throat culture. As shown here on the left, the colonies are nonhemolytic after overnight incubation, compared with the strong beta hemolysis of group A streptococci. *Arcanobacterium* was previously included in the genus *Corynebacterium*, but it is catalase-negative. Microscopically, these gram-positive bacilli resemble *Corynebacterium* spp. **B,** Colonies of *Arcanobacterium haemolyticum* (*top*) and *Streptococcus pyogenes* (*bottom*) (close-up after overnight incubation).

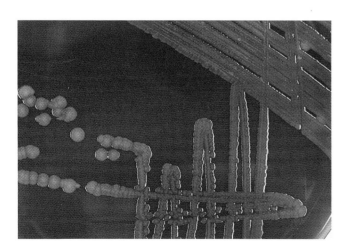

**7-22 Colonies of** *Rhodococcus* **on 5% sheep** **blood agar.** *Rhodococcus* is classified within the "nocardio-forms" group. *Rhodococcus equi* was also previously included in the genus *Corynebacterium* as well as the genus *Mycobacterium*. The microorganism grows well on sheep blood agar, and colonies can resemble *Klebsiella*, but it does not grow on MacConkey agar. Colonies usually develop a pink pigment after prolonged incubation.

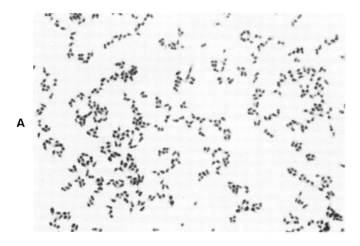

A

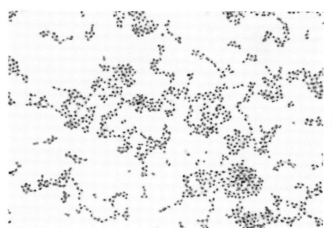

B

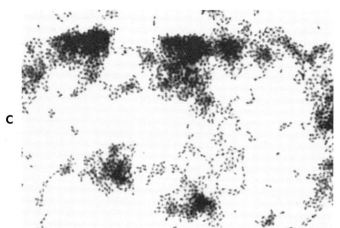

C

**7-23 A, B, Microscopic appearance of *Rhodococcus* sp. (×1250).** Young cells from colonies less than 24 hours old appear elongated (**A**) and may even appear rodlike. **B,** Cellular morphology changes to a more coccoid form within 24 to 48 hours. Mature forms may even be filamentous. Branched filaments may fragment into rods and cocci during the growth cycle. **C, Modified Kinyoun acid-fast stain.** *Rhodococcus equi* may be partially acid-fast when stained with a modified Kinyoun stain using 2% $H_2SO_4$ as the decolorizing agent.

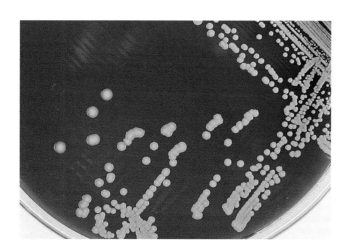

**7-24 Colonies of *Oerskovia* spp. on 5% sheep blood agar.** *Oerskovia* are motile gram-positive filaments that fragment into rodlike forms. This microorganism can be presumptively identified by its microscopic morphology, motility, hydrolysis of esculin, and yellow pigment on sheep blood agar.

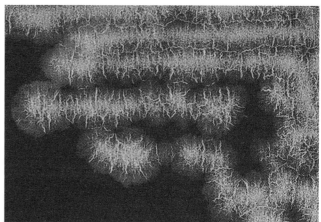

**7-25 Very young colonies of *Oerskovia* on 5% sheep blood agar (×10).** *Oerskovia* previously belonged to the unnamed coryneform bacteria of Centers for Disease Control (CDC) group A. They are characterized by colonies with a filamentous appearance that is observed with a light microscope under low power.

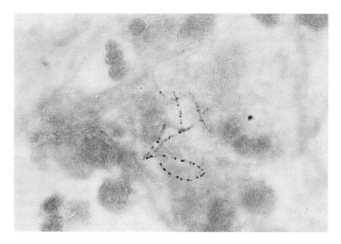

**7-26 Gram stain *Nocardia* spp. (×1250).** *Nocardia* species are branching, beaded, filamentous gram-positive bacilli, approximately 1 μm in diameter. They can also appear as coccoid or coccobacillary forms. Care should be taken when examining the slides because of the faint staining properties of these microorganisms and other actinomycetes.

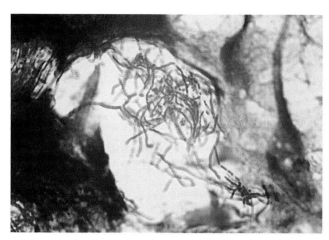

**7-27 Modified Kinyoun acid-fast stain.** *Nocardia* species appear acid-fast when stained with a modified Kinyoun stain using 2% H$_2$SO$_4$ as the decolorizing agent. This feature helps to distinguish this microorganism from other actinomycetes.

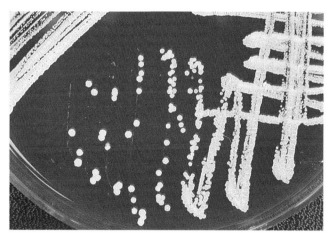

**7-28 Colonies of *Nocardia asteroides* on 5% sheep blood agar.** Colonies initially appear as powdery, and as they mature they can develop a number of colors, ranging from a chalky-white to yellow-orange, buff, red, purple, brown, and black. Most colonies have an earthy odor.

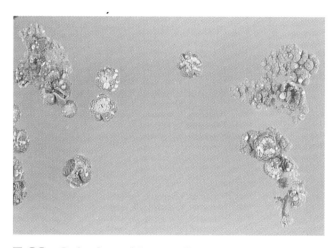

**7-29 Colonies of *Nocardia asteroides* on BAY agar plate.** Yellow-orange colonies of *Nocardia asteroides.* The yellow color is more common with colonies of most *Nocardia* spp.

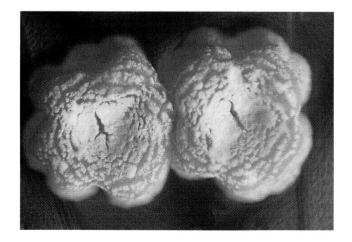

**7-30 Colonies of *Nocardia asteroides* growing on BAY plate (×15).** Colonies are large, dry, bumpy, and heaped after 9 days incubation at 27°C. This morphology has been referred to as glabrous orange form.

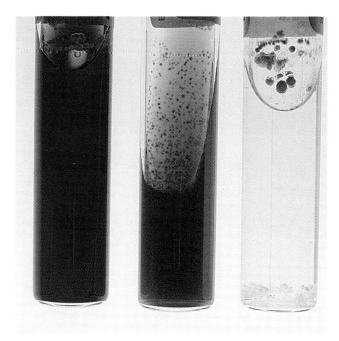

**7-31 Identification of the genus *Nocardia* with biochemical reactions.** *Nocardia* spp. are aerobic actinomycetes that reduce nitrate to nitrite (*tube on left*), hydrolyze urea (*tube in center*), and grow on the surface of a broth medium, such as the thioglycolate broth on the right.

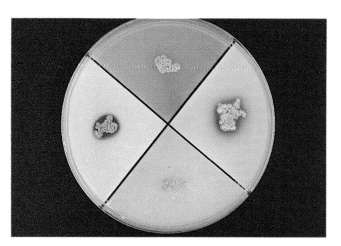

**7-32 Amino acid hydrolysis reactions of *Nocardia brasiliensis.*** Identification to the species level is usually made on the basis of hydrolysis of amino acids: casein, tyrosine, xanthine, and hypoxanthine. Clearing of the agar around the colony is interpreted as a positive reaction. Both casein and tyrosine are positive (*left and right quadrants*) on this plate. Xanthine and hypoxanthine (*top and bottom quadrants*) are negative.

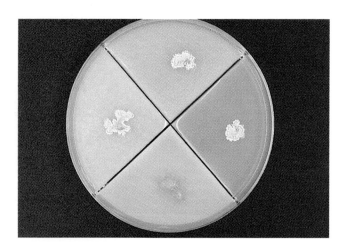

**7-33 Amino acid hydrolysis reactions of *Nocardia asteroides.*** All amino acid reactions are negative on this identification plate; casein, tyrosine, xanthine, and hypoxanthine.

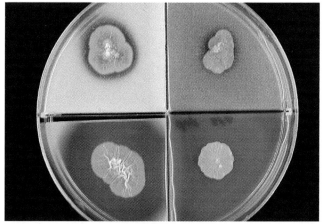

**7-34 Amino acid hydrolysis reactions of *Streptomyces* spp.** All reactions are positive on this identification plate. Unlike any *Nocardia* spp., *Streptomyces* spp. hydrolyze casein, tyrosine, xanthine, and hypoxanthine. Colonial morphology resembles the chalky, dry white colonies of *Nocardia* spp. Although *Streptomyces* spp. are urea-positive, they are nitrate-negative, distinguishing the genera from *Nocardia* spp.

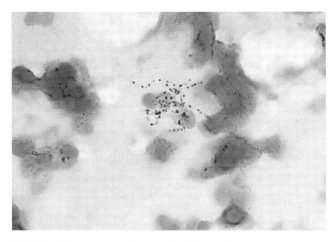

**7-35 Gram stain of *Streptomyces* spp. (×1250).** *Streptomyces* spp. are characterized microscopically by branching, beaded, gram-positive filamentous bacilli, indistinguishable from *Nocardia* spp. Unlike *Nocardia* spp., the partial acid-fast stain is negative.

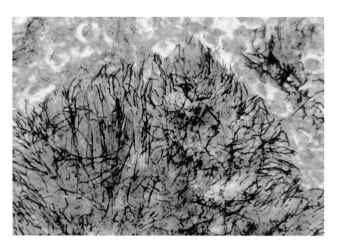

**7-36 Gomori methenamine silver stain of *Actinomyces* spp. (×1250).** The slide was prepared from a tissue biopsy specimen. In the center is a characteristic "sulfur granule," which consists of a granular microcolony surrounded by purulent exudate. The *Actinomyces* spp. are gram-positive bacilli that vary in size from short, diphtheroid forms to long, branching filaments. Unlike *Nocardia* spp. they are not partially acid-fast.

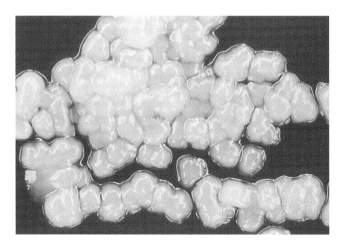

**7-37 Colonies of *Actinomyces* spp. (×10).** These are the characteristic "molar tooth" colonies of *Actinomyces israelii* that develop in 1 to 2 weeks on agar plates incubated under anaerobic conditions. These colonies are heaped and raised with irregular margins.

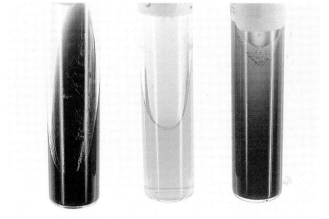

**7-38 Biochemical identification of *Actinomyces israelii*.** Most *Actinomyces* spp. reduce nitrate to nitrite (*red colored broth on right*) including *Actinomyces israelii*. Additionally, *Actinomyces israelii* hydrolyzes esculin (*black slant on left*), but not urea (*yellow slant in center*).

# CHAPTER 8 *Enterobacteriaceae*

The *Enterobacteriaceae* are the most common bacterial isolates encountered in the diagnostic laboratory. They can be isolated from a wide variety of specimens either as normal flora (predominantly in the intestinal tract) or pathogens. The gram-negative bacillary microscopic morphology is similar among all species. Colonies are usually large and gray on 5% sheep blood agar. Rapid lactose fermenters appear pink on MacConkey agar and have a greenish metallic sheen on Eosin methylene blue (EMB). The *Enterobacteriaceae* are very active biochemically and can be identified with a wide variety of tests. Four characteristics of the *Enterobacteriaceae* are growth on MacConkey agar, oxidase-negative, glucose fermentation, and reduction of nitrates to nitrites.

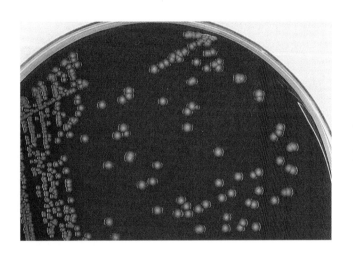

**8-1 *Enterobacteriaceae* on 5% sheep blood agar.** Characteristic colonial morphology on 5% sheep blood agar showing large, dull, gray, nonhemolytic colonies. Hemolysis is variable and not characteristic of any one genus.

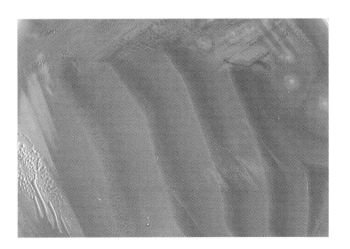

**8-2 *Proteus* species on 5% sheep blood agar.** Growth appears to spread as a film on the plate from the original colony or streak line, often extending in waves. This characteristic of *Proteus* spp. is called swarming and suggests that the microorganism is motile by means of flagella.

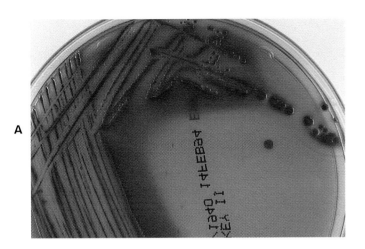

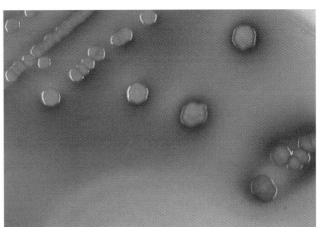

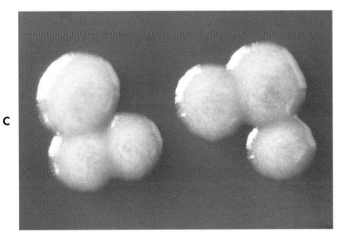

**8-3 A,** *E. coli* **on MacConkey agar.** Rapid lactose fermenting strains of *E. coli* appear as shiny pink colonies on MacConkey agar. **B,** *E. coli* **on MacConkey agar (close-up). C,** *E. coli* **on 5% sheep blood agar (close-up).** Colonies are shiny, opaque, cream-colored, and attain 2 to 4 mm diameter overnight.

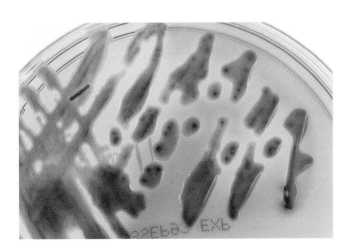

**8-4** *Klebsiella pneumoniae* **on MacConkey agar.** Rapid lactose fermenting colonies of *Klebsiella pneumoniae* appears pink, large, glistening, and mucoid. This strain is probably encapsulated and therefore appears mucoid. Although this appearance is associated with *Klebsiella pneumoniae*, it is not unique for that species.

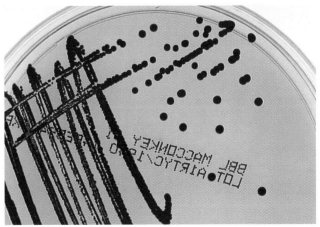

**8-5 Pigmented** *Serratia* **sp. on MacConkey agar.** These colonies appear red and should not be confused with the pink color due to lactose fermentation shown in 8-3. Rare strains of *Serratia* spp. produce pigment, which is seen on all solid media including the blood agar plate.

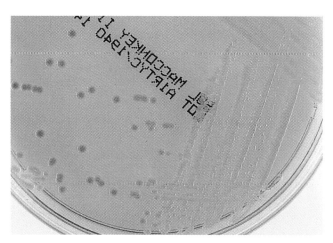

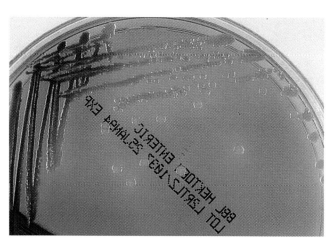

**8-6** *Enterobacteriaceae* **on MacConkey agar.**
All late lactose fermenters and lactose-negative species of the *Enterobacteriaceae* appear as colorless (color of the medium) colonies on MacConkey. The colonies of the late lactose fermenting species may appear faintly pink after 48 to 72 hours of incubation.

**8-7** *Enterobacteriaceae* **on Hektoen enteric agar (HE).** Most species of *Enterobacteriaceae*, except for the rapid lactose fermenters including some *Escherichia, Klebsiella, Enterobacter,* and *Citrobacter* species, appear colorless on either MacConkey or eosin methylene blue (EMB) agars. Fecal specimens should be inoculated onto a more selective medium such as HE agar or xylose-lysine-desoxycholate (XLD) agar to help differentiate enteric intestinal pathogens. Fermentation of lactose, sucrose, and/or salicin results in yellow or salmon colored colonies due to the pH change on the bromthymol blue and acid fuchsin indicators.

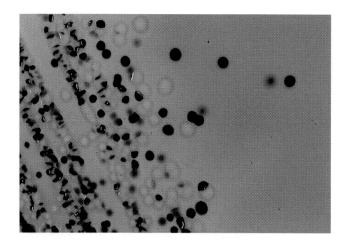

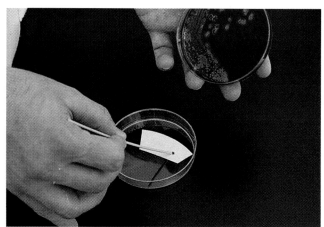

**8-8** *Salmonella* **spp. and other** *Enterobacteriaceae* **on Hektoen enteric agar.** If an organism does not ferment lactose, sucrose, or salicin, the colonies will appear green (color of the medium). If the microorganism produces H$_2$S, an important characteristic of the *Enterobacteriaceae*, the colonies will have black centers and will appear completely black with prolonged incubation. These black colonies are characteristic of most *Salmonella* spp. on HE agar.

**8-9** **Identification of the** *Enterobacteriaceae* **by the rapid spot test method.** Spot tests are commonly used for the rapid, presumptive identification of many microorganism groups. For this method, filter paper or a paper disk is impregnated with the substrate. To perform the test, one or more colonies are selected with a sterile wooden applicator stick from the described medium and applied to the test surface.

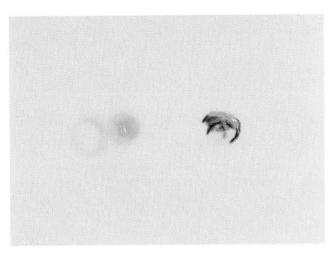

**8-10 Oxidase spot test.** Some microorganisms possess either cytochrome oxidase or indophenol oxidase, which catalyze the transport of electrons from donor compounds (NADH) to electron receptors ($O_2$). In this test, the substrate paraphenylenediamine dihydrochloride serves as an artificial electron acceptor for the enzyme oxidase. The dye is oxidized and forms the colored compound, indophenol blue. For this test, filter paper is saturated with the substrate. Colonies of the microrganism to be tested are rubbed onto the filter paper with a sterile wooden applicator stick. An immediate color change to a deep blue indicates a positive test result (*spot on the right*). The *Enterobacteriaceae* are oxidase-negative and therefore the inoculum should not change the color of the paper (*spot on the left*).

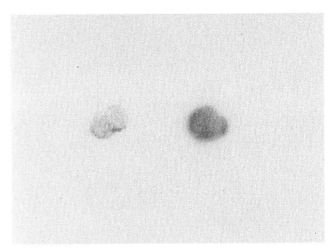

**8-11 Indole spot test.** Indole is one of the degradation products of the amino acid tryptophan. Indole produced by a microorganism grown in a medium that is rich in tryptophan can be detected by its ability to combine with certain aldehydes to form a colored compound. For the spot test, filter paper is soaked with either paradimethylaminocinnamaldehyde or paradimethylaminobenzaldehyde (Kovacs reagent). Colonies of the microorganism to be tested are rubbed onto the filter paper with a sterile wooden applicator stick. If paradimethylaminocinnamaldehyde is used, a blue-green color appears immediately in the presence of indole. If Kovacs reagent is used, a bright pink-red color develops. In this figure, using filter paper soaked with paradimethylaminocinnamaldehyde, the colony on the right is positive while the one on the left is negative. The pink color is the result of a lactose-positive color selected from MacConkey agar.

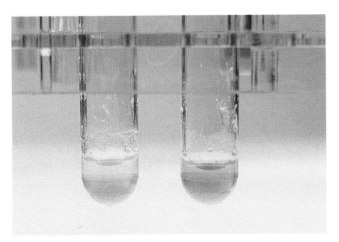

**8-12 o-nitrophenyl-β-D-galactopyranoside (ONPG) test.** The enzyme β-galactosidase mediates lactose fermentation. Rapid lactose fermenters, however, possess a permease enzyme that speeds the reaction, yielding pink colonies on MacConkey agar. Production of β-galactosidase only results in delayed lactose fermentation (2 to 10 days). True nonlactose fermenters possess neither enzyme. The ONPG test is a rapid test (4 hours) for β-galactosidase. β-galactosidase breaks down the substrate ONPG into o-nitrophenyl, a yellow compound, and galactose. A yellow color indicates a positive test (*right tube*) and no color change (negative) indicates a true nonlactose fermenter (*left tube*).

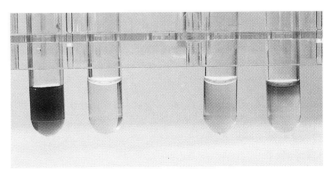

**8-13 Methyl red—Voges-Proskauer (MRVP) test.** Both tests are performed from the same inoculum suspension, which is divided for testing. The methyl red test is used to determine the pH of the end products of glucose fermentation. In converting glucose to pyruvic acid, some *Enterobacteriaceae* produce acid end products (pH less than 4.4), which turn the methyl red indicator red, while others produce acetoin (pH greater than 6.0), which turns the indicator yellow. The Voges-Proskauer test detects acetoin. The reagents α-naphthol and KOH are added to the broth suspension. Acetoin is oxidized to diacetyl, yielding a red color (pH greater than 6.0). The left set of tubes shows a positive MR and a negative VP (no color change), and the right set shows a negative MR and a positive VP.

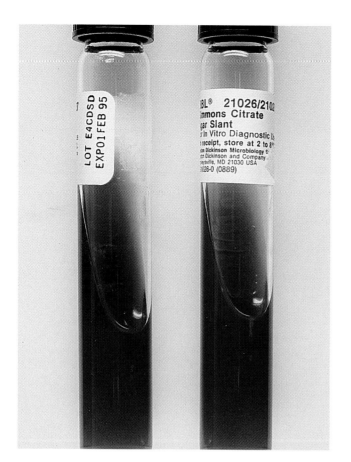

**8-14   Citrate utilization test.** Some of the *Enterobacteriaceae* have the ability to utilize citrate as a sole source of carbon. In this test, a colony is inoculated onto the surface of a citrate slant and the medium is incubated overnight at 35°C. The medium contains sodium citrate, ammonium salts, and bromthymol blue indicator. The presence of a blue color indicates the presence of alkaline end products and a positive citrate test (*left tube*). If the test is negative there is no color change (*right tube*).

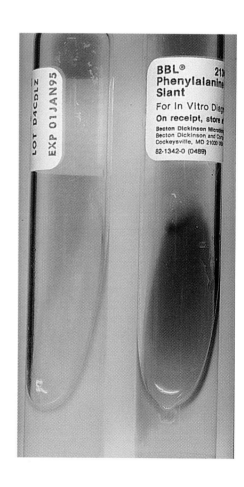

**8-15   Phenylalanine deaminase (PAD) test**. This test is based on the principle that some microorganisms can remove an amine group from the amino acid phenylalanine, resulting in the production of phenylpyruvic acid. A microorganism growing on a phenylalanine agar slant is tested by adding a few drops of a 10% ferric chloride solution. A green color (*right tube*) indicates a positive test result. The slant remains colorless with a negative test result (*left tube*). This test is helpful in differentiating the tribe: *Proteae* (PAD-positive) from the other *Enterobacteriaceae* (PAD-negative).

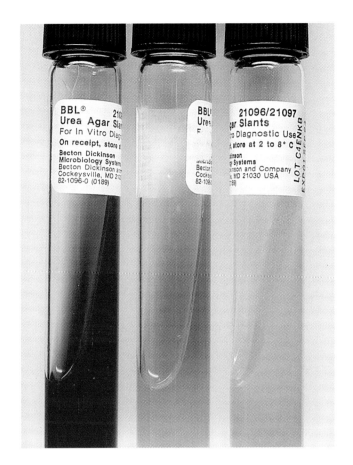

**8-16  Urease test.** Microorganisms that possess the enzyme urease hydrolyze urea to ammonia and $CO_2$. The phenol red indicator turns cerise (dark pink) in the presence of the alkaline end products. This figure shows three inoculated Christensen's urea slants that were incubated overnight. The left and middle tubes are positive. The left tube was inoculated with *Proteus mirabilis,* a rapid urea hydrolyzer (2 to 4 hours), the middle tube was inoculated with *Klebsiella pneumoniae,* a slow urea hydrolyzer (18 to 24 hours), and the right tube was inoculated with *E. coli,* a urease-negative microorganism.

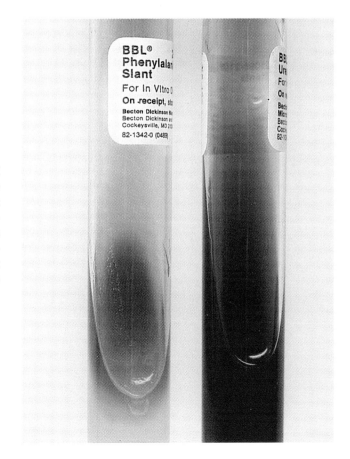

**8-17  Positive PAD and urea tests.** Four species of the *Enterobacteriaceae* are PAD and urea-positive: *Proteus mirabilis, Proteus vulgaris, Morganella morganii,* and *Providencia rettgeri.* If the isolate tested produced these reactions and also swarmed on blood agar, it would be a *Proteus* spp. A spot indole test would identify the species; *Proteus mirabilis* is indole-negative and *Proteus vulgaris* is indole-positive. The citrate test would differentiate the nonswarmers; *Morganella morganii* is citrate-negative and *Providencia rettgeri* is citrate-positive.

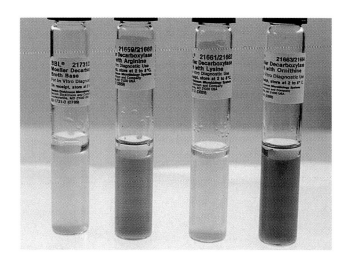

**8-18    Decarboxylase-dihydrolase tests.** The decarboxylase enzyme removes carboxyl groups from the amino acids lysine and ornithine. The dihydrolase enzyme removes a carboxyl group from arginine. Glucose base without the amino acid (*left tube; control*) and tubes containing glucose plus the amino acid substrates are inoculated. Decarboxylation and dihydrolation are anaerobic reactions, so the inoculated tubes must be overlaid with sterile mineral oil to exclude air. Initially, all broths turn yellow due to acidification of the indicator (bromcresol purple) by the acid end products of glucose fermentation. If the amino acid is decarboxylated, the alkaline end product causes the indicator to revert to an alkaline pH (purple). In this figure, arginine (second from left) and ornithine (right tube) are positive and lysine is negative.

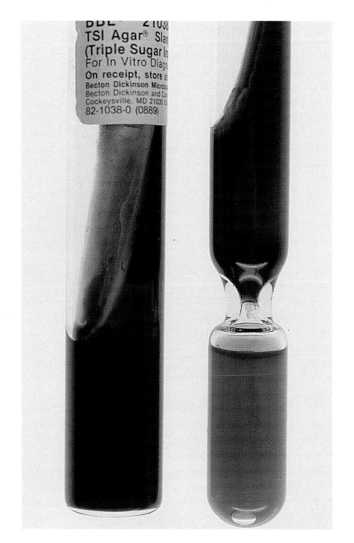

**8-19    Triple Sugar Iron (TSI) agar slant and r/b₁ tube.** TSI agar detects fermentation of glucose, lactose and sucrose, $H_2S$ production, and gas formation. The medium contains one part glucose to 10 parts lactose and sucrose, ferric ammonium citrate, and phenol red indicator. If the microorganism ferments glucose alone, the entire tube (slant and butt) will turn acid (yellow); however, the microorganism will begin to degrade proteins on the agar surface, resulting in alkaline end products and a pink slant. If lactose and/or sucrose are fermented, the entire tube remains yellow because of the greater concentration of these carbohydrates. $H_2S$ reacts with ferric ammonium citrate to produce a black end product, ferrous sulfide. Gas formation is detected by the presence of bubbles or cracks in the agar. The **r/b₁ tube** (Remel Laboratories, Lenexa, Kan.) is a manual commercial identification system. Five reactions can occur in the upper portion of the first tube: glucose and lactose fermentation, $H_2S$ production, gas formation, and phenylalanine deamination. Lysine decarboxylation occurs in the lower (anaerobic) portion. In this example, glucose is fermented and $H_2S$ is produced in the TSI (*left side*). The yellow color indicating glucose fermentation is masked by the black end product of $H_2S$ production. The same reaction appears in the upper portion of the r/b₁ tube; lysine is positive in the lower portion. This reaction suggests *Salmonella* spp.

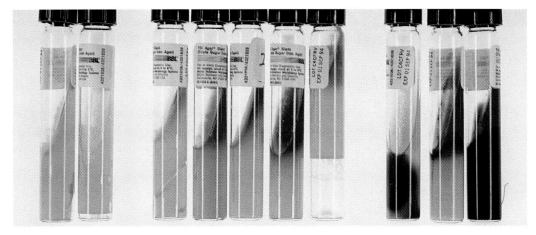

**8-20  TSI slant reactions.** The 10 TSI tubes have the following reactions* (*left to right*):

|      | Slant    | Butt | H₂S    | Gas formation |
|------|----------|------|--------|---------------|
| #1   | acid     | acid | 0      | 0             |
| #2   | acid     | acid | 0      | +             |
| #3   | alkaline | acid | 0      | +             |
| #4   | alkaline | acid | 0      | 0             |
| #5   | alkaline | acid | 0      | 0             |
| #6   | alkaline | acid | 0      | 0             |
| #7   | alkaline | acid | 0      | +             |
| #8   | acid     | acid | +      | 0             |
| #9   | alkaline | acid | slight | 0             |
| #10  | alkaline | acid | +      | +             |

*Acid = yellow; alkaline = red; $H_2S$-positive = black; gas = cracks, bubbles.

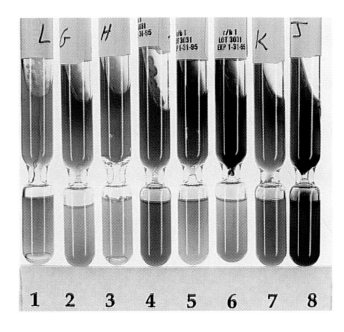

**8-21  r/b₁ reactions.** The eight r/b₁ tubes have the following reactions*:

|      | Slant    | Butt | H₂S    | Gas formation | PAD | Lysine |
|------|----------|------|--------|---------------|-----|--------|
| #1   | acid     | acid | 0      | +             | 0   | 0      |
| #2   | alkaline | acid | 0      | 0             | 0   | 0      |
| #3   | alkaline | acid | 0      | +             | 0   | 0      |
| #4   | alkaline | acid | 0      | 0             | 0   | +      |
| #5   | alkaline | acid | 0      | 0             | +   | 0      |
| #6   | alkaline | acid | +      | 0             | +   | 0      |
| #7   | alkaline | acid | slight | 0             | 0   | +      |
| #8   | alkaline | acid | +      | +             | 0   | +      |

*Acid = yellow; alkaline = red; $H_2S$-positive = black; gas = cracks, bubbles; PAD positive = brown; lysine-positive = red.

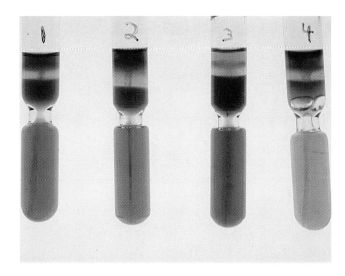

**8-22   r/b₂ medium and reactions.** This tube has an upper (aerobic) and lower (anaerobic) portion. Indole is interpreted in the upper portion and ornithine decarboxylase and motility are interpreted in the lower portion. This tube is similar to the conventional MIO (motility-indole-ornithine) medium.

The four r/b₂ tubes shown have the following reactions*:

|     | Motility | Indole | Ornithine |
|-----|----------|--------|-----------|
| #1  | +        | +      | +         |
| #2  | 0        | +      | +         |
| #3  | +        | 0      | +         |
| #4  | 0        | +      | 0         |

*Indole-positive=red (+) at the surface of the top portion, ornithine positive=purple red, motility positive=turbid medium with a hazy stab line

**8-23   CIT/RHAM medium and reactions.** The upper (aerobic) portion of this medium is for demonstration of citrate utilization, and the lower (anaerobic) portion is to detect rhamnose fermentation.

The four CIT/RHAM tubes have the following reactions*:

|     | Citrate | Rhamnose |
|-----|---------|----------|
| #1  | 0       | 0        |
| #2  | 0       | +        |
| #3  | +       | +        |
| #4  | +       | 0        |

*Citrate-positive = blue; citrate-negative = green; rhamnose-positive = yellow; rhamnose-negative = green.

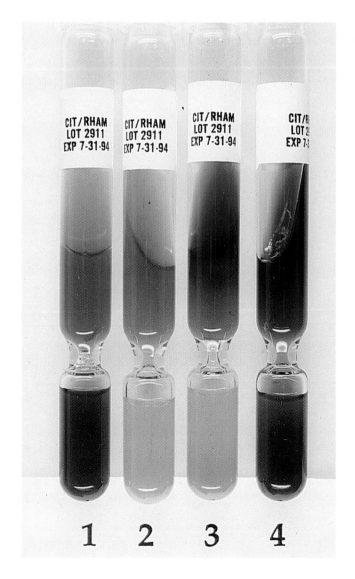

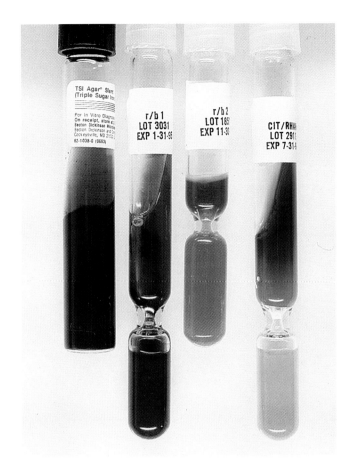

**8-24** **Characteristic reactions of** *Salmonella* **spp. (except Salmonella typhi)**

| TSI | r/b₁ | r/b₂ | CIT/RHAM |
|-----|------|------|----------|
| alk/acid | alk/acid | ornithine + | +/+ |
| H₂S+ | H₂S + | motile | |
| | lysine + | indole 0 | |
| | PAD 0 | | |

**8-25** **Characteristic reactions of** *Salmonella typhi.*

| TSI | r/b₁ | r/b₂ | CIT/RHAM |
|-----|------|------|----------|
| alk/acid | alk/acid | ornithine 0 | 0/0 |
| slight H₂S + | slight H₂S + | motile | |
| | lysine + | indole 0 | |
| | PAD 0 | | |

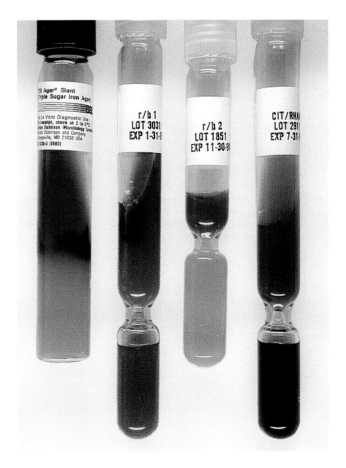

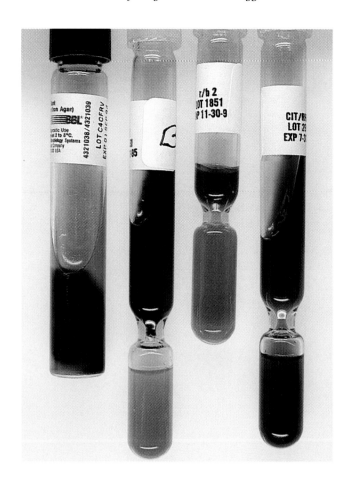

**8-26 Characteristic reactions of *Proteus vulgaris*.**

| TSI | r/b₁ | r/b₂ | CIT/RHAM |
|---|---|---|---|
| acid/acid | alk/acid | ornithine 0 | +/0 |
| H₂S + | H₂S + | motile | |
| | PAD + | Indole + | |
| | lysine 0 | | |

**8-27 Characteristic reactions of *Yersinia enterocolitica*.**

| TSI | r/b₁ | r/b₂ | CIT/RHAM |
|---|---|---|---|
| alk/acid | alk/acid | ornithine + | 0/+ |
| H₂S 0 | lysine 0 | non motile | |
| | H₂S 0 | Indole + | |
| | PAD 0 | | |

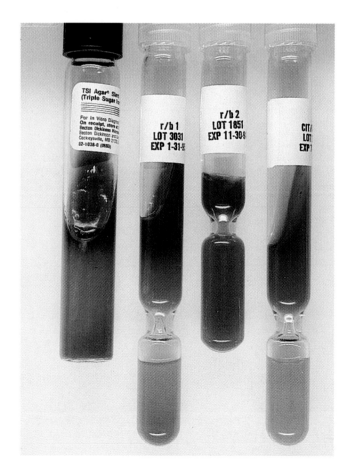

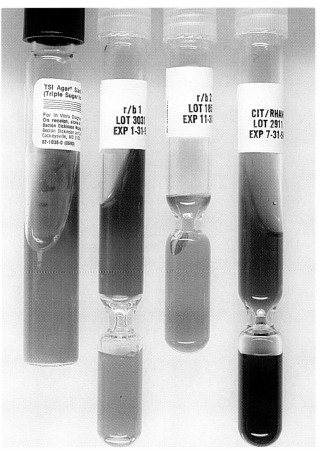

**8-28 Characteristic reactions of *Shigella* spp.**

| TSI | r/b₁ | r/b₂ | CIT/RHAM |
|---|---|---|---|
| alk/acid | alk/acid | ornithine 0 | 0/0 |
| H₂S 0 | lysine 0 | nonmotile | |
| | H₂S 0 | indole 0 | |
| | PAD 0 | | |

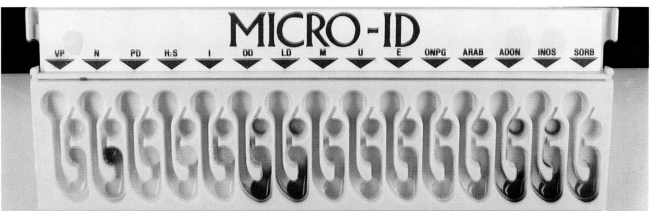

**8-29 Characteristic reactions of *E. coli* using MICRO-ID strip.** The MICRO-ID (Organon Teknika, Durham, N.C.) strip contains 15 biochemical tests for the rapid identification (4 hours) of the *Enterobacteriaceae*. The system is based on the principle that the heavy inoculum suspension of the organism to be tested contains high levels of preformed enzymes. The tests included in the system are Voges-Proskauer (VP), nitrate (N), phenylalanine deaminase (PD), H₂S, indole (I), ornithine (OD) and lysine decarboxylase (LD), malonate (M), urea (U), esculin (E), ONPG, arabinose (ARAB), adonitol (ADON), inositol (INOS), and sorbitol (SORB). The test results are interpreted visually, coded numerically, and compared to identification tables or the MICRO-ID profile code book to make the identification. The interpretation of this example is:

| VP | N | PD | H₂S | I | OD | LD | M | U | E | ONPG | | ARAB | ADON | INOS | SORB |
|---|---|---|---|---|---|---|---|---|---|---|---|---|---|---|---|
| 0 | + | 0 | 0 | + | + | + | 0 | 0 | 0 | + | | + | 0 | 0 | 0 |

The identification is *E. coli* and the profile code number is 23430. The code was derived by dividing the tests into 5 groups of three and assigning a score to each. The first test of each set is given a score of 4, the second test is assigned a 2 and the third test is assigned a 1. If any of the tests are positive, it is given its score, but it receives a 0 if it is negative. The numbers in a set can range from 0 to 7.

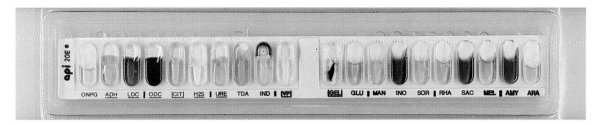

**8-30 Characteristic reactions of *E. coli* using the API 20 E strip.** The API 20E strip (bioMerieux Vitek, Hazelwood, Mo.) is a self-contained system of 20 microtubes of dehydrated substrates, a miniaturized version of conventional procedures, designed for overnight incubation. Identification is made by adding necessary reagents and then visually interpreting the results. The tests included in the system are: ONPG, arginine dihydrolase (ADC), lysine (LDC) and ornithine (ODC) decarboxylase, citrate (CIT), $H_2S$, urea (URE), tryptophan deaminase (TDA), indole (IND), Voges-Proskauer (VP), gelatin (GEL), glucose (GLU), mannitol (MAN), inositol (INO), sorbitol (SOR), rhamnose (RHA), sucrose (SAC), melibiose (MEL), amygdalin (AMY), and arabinose (ARA). An oxidase test must be performed separately. Numerical coding of results allows computerized interpretation of patterns, lists of which are available in a codebook or in computerized form. The interpretation of this example is:

| ONPG | ADC | LDC | ODC | CIT | $H_2S$ | URE | TDA | IND | VP | | GEL | GLU | MAN | INO | SOR | RHA | SAC | MEL | AMY | ARA |
|---|---|---|---|---|---|---|---|---|---|---|---|---|---|---|---|---|---|---|---|---|
| + | 0 | + | + | 0 | 0 | 0 | 0 | + | 0 | | 0 | + | + | 0 | + | + | 0 | + | 0 | + |

The identification is *E. coli* and the profile code number is 5144552. The code was derived by dividing the tests into 7 groups of three (oxidase reaction is the third test in the last set) and assigning a score to each. The first test of each set is given a 1, the second test is assigned a 2 and the third test is assigned a 4. If any of the tests are positive, it is given its score and receives a 0 if it is negative. The total scores in a set can range from 0 to 7.

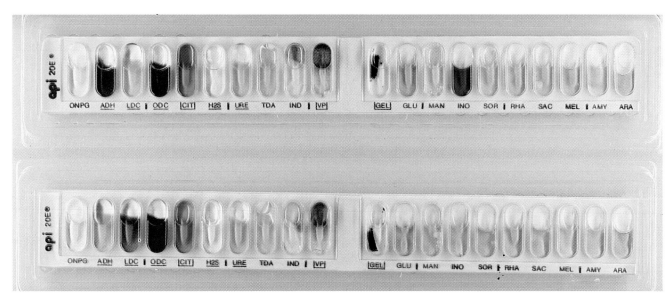

**8-31 Characteristic reactions of *Enterobacter aerogenes* (top) and *Enterobacter cloacae* (bottom) using API 20 E strips.** The interpretation of these tests in this example is:

| | ONPG | ADC | LDC | ODC | CIT | $H_2S$ | URE | TDA | IND | V P | | | GEL | GLU | MAN | INO | SOR | RHA | SAC | MEL | AMY | ARA |
|---|---|---|---|---|---|---|---|---|---|---|---|---|---|---|---|---|---|---|---|---|---|---|
| E clo | + | + | 0 | + | + | 0 | 0 | 0 | 0 | + | | E clo | 0 | + | + | 0 | + | + | + | + | + | + |
| E aer | + | 0 | + | + | + | 0 | 0 | 0 | 0 | + | | E aer | 0 | + | + | + | + | + | + | + | + | + |

The profile code number for *E. cloacae* (E clo) is 3305573.
The profile code number for *E. aerogenes* (E aer) is 5305773.
The major differences between the two species are the reactions with arginine, lysine, and inositol.

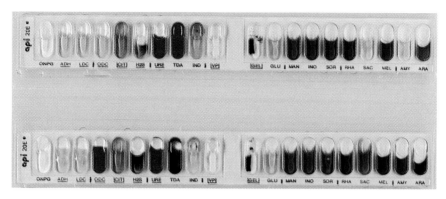

**8-32 Characteristic reactions of *Proteus mirabilis* (top) and *Proteus vulgaris* (bottom) using API 20 E strips.** The interpretation of these tests in this example is:

|       | ONPG | ADC | LDC | ODC | CIT | H₂S | URE | TDA | IND | V P |
|-------|------|-----|-----|-----|-----|-----|-----|-----|-----|-----|
| P vul | 0    | 0   | 0   | 0   | +   | +   | +   | +   | +   | 0   |
| P mir | 0    | 0   | 0   | +   | +   | +   | +   | +   | 0   | 0   |

|       | GEL | GLU | MAN | INO | SOR | RHA | SAC | MEL | AMY | ARA |
|-------|-----|-----|-----|-----|-----|-----|-----|-----|-----|-----|
| P vul | 0   | +   | 0   | 0   | 0   | 0   | +   | 0   | +   | 0   |
| P mir | 0   | +   | 0   | 0   | 0   | 0   | 0   | 0   | 0   | 0   |

The profile code number for *P. vulgaris* (P vul) is 0674021.

The profile code number for *P. mirabilis* (P mir) is 0734000.

The differences between the two species are the reactions with ornithine, indole, sucrose, and amygdalin.

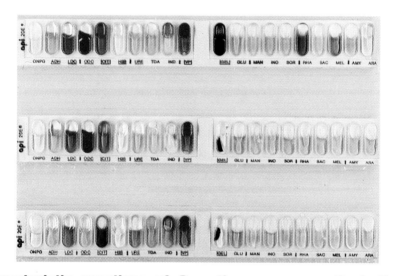

**8-33 Characteristic reactions of *Serratia marcescens* (top), *Enterobacter aerogenes* (middle), and *Klebsiella oxytoca* (bottom) using API 20 E strips.**

|       | ONPG | ADC | LDC | ODC | CIT | H₂S | URE | TDA | IND | V P |
|-------|------|-----|-----|-----|-----|-----|-----|-----|-----|-----|
| S mar | +    | 0   | +   | +   | +   | 0   | 0   | 0   | 0   | +   |
| E aer | +    | 0   | +   | +   | +   | 0   | 0   | 0   | 0   | +   |
| K oxy | +    | 0   | +   | 0   | +   | 0   | 0   | 0   | +   | +   |

|       | GEL | GLU | MAN | INO | SOR | RHA | SAC | MEL | AMY | ARA |
|-------|-----|-----|-----|-----|-----|-----|-----|-----|-----|-----|
| S mar | +   | +   | +   | +   | +   | 0   | +   | 0   | +   | +   |
| E aer | 0   | +   | +   | +   | +   | +   | +   | +   | +   | +   |
| K oxy | 0   | +   | +   | +   | +   | +   | +   | +   | +   | +   |

The profile code number for *Serratia marcescens* (S mar) is 5307723.

The profile code number for *E. aerogenes* (E aer) is 5305773.

The profile code number for *Klebsiella oxytoca* (K oxy) is 5245773.

The differences between *S. marcescens* and *E. aerogenes* are the reactions with gelatin, rhamnose, and melibiose.

The differences between *K. oxytoca* and *E. aerogenes* are the reactions with ornithine and indole.

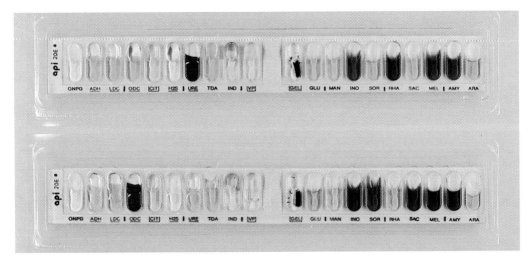

**8-34 Characteristic reactions of *Yersinia enterocolitica* and *Shigella sonnei* using API 20 E strips.**

|       | ONPG  | ADC | LDC | ODC | CIT | H₂S | URE | TDA | IND | V P |
|-------|-------|-----|-----|-----|-----|-----|-----|-----|-----|-----|
| Y ent | w+/0  | 0   | 0   | 0   | 0   | 0   | +   | 0   | 0   | 0   |
| S son | w+/0  | 0   | 0   | +   | 0   | 0   | 0   | 0   | 0   | 0   |

|       | GEL | GLU | MAN | INO | SOR | RHA | SAC | MEL | AMY | ARA |
|-------|-----|-----|-----|-----|-----|-----|-----|-----|-----|-----|
| Y ent | 0   | +   | +   | 0   | +   | 0   | +   | 0   | 0   | +   |
| S son | 0   | +   | +   | 0   | 0   | +   | 0   | 0   | 0   | +   |

The profile code number for *Yersinia enterocolitica* (Y ent) is 1014522.

The profile code number for *Shigella sonnei* (S son) is 1104112.

The differences between the two species are the reactions with ornithine, urea, sorbitol, rhamnose, and sucrose.

w = weak positive.

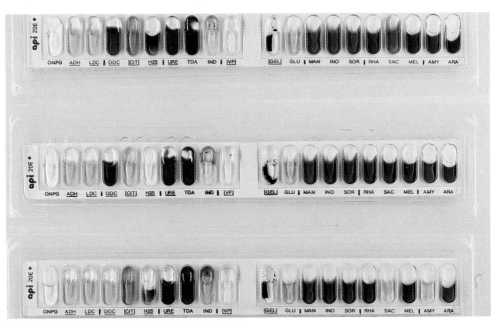

**8-35 Characteristic reactions of *Proteus mirabilis* (top), *Morganella morganii* (middle), and *Proteus vulgaris* (bottom) using API 20 E strips.**

|       | ONPG | ADC | LDC | ODC | CIT | H₂S | URE | TDA | IND | V P |
|-------|------|-----|-----|-----|-----|-----|-----|-----|-----|-----|
| P mir | 0    | 0   | 0   | +   | +   | +   | +   | +   | 0   | 0   |
| M mor | 0    | 0   | 0   | +   | 0   | 0   | +   | +   | +   | 0   |
| P vul | 0    | 0   | 0   | 0   | +   | +   | +   | +   | +   | 0   |

|       | GEL | GLU | MAN | INO | SOR | RHA | SAC | MEL | AMY | ARA |
|-------|-----|-----|-----|-----|-----|-----|-----|-----|-----|-----|
| P mir | 0   | +   | 0   | 0   | 0   | 0   | 0   | 0   | 0   | 0   |
| M mor | 0   | +   | 0   | 0   | 0   | 0   | 0   | 0   | 0   | 0   |
| P vul | 0   | +   | 0   | 0   | 0   | 0   | +   | 0   | +   | 0   |

The profile code number for *P. mirabilis* (P mir) is 0734000.

The profile code number for *M. morganii* (M mor) is 0174000.

The profile code number for *P. vulgaris* (P vul) is 0674021.

The differences between *M. morganii* and *P. mirabilis* are the reactions with citrate, H₂S, and indole.

The differences between *M. morganii* and *P. vulgaris* are the reactions with ornithine, citrate, H₂S, sucrose, and amygdalin.

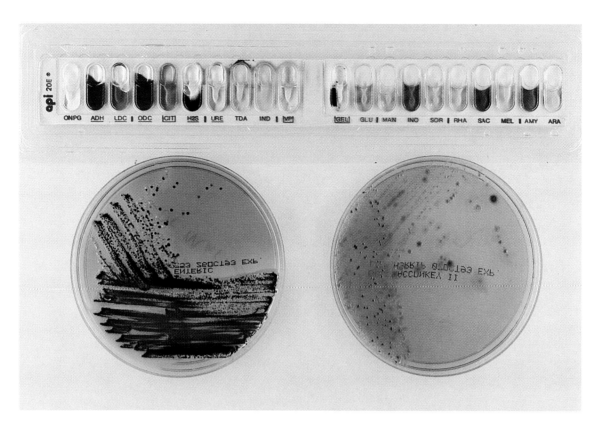

**8-36  Comparing colonial morphology with biochemical identification.** An important step in the final identification of an isolate is to compare the biochemical reaction with the colonial morphology and reactions on the primary plating media. In this example, the colonies of *Salmonella* spp. are H₂S-positive on the HE agar and the H₂S is also positive on the API 20 E.

# CHAPTER 9 Other Gram-Negative Microorganisms

T he gram-negative microorganisms presented in this section are those that are not in the family *Enterobacteriaceae*. Included are the *Neisseria* and *Moraxella* species, miscellaneous fastidious gram-negative bacilli (*Haemophilus, Bordetella, Brucella, Pasteurella, Eikenella, Kingella,* and *Capnocytophaga* spp.), the curved or comma-shaped gram-negative bacilli (*Campylobacter* and *Vibrio* spp.), and the nonfermentative gram-negative bacilli (*Pseudomonas, Sphingomonas, Stenotrophomonas, Shewanella, Acinetobacter,* and *Flavobacterium* spp.).

## *Neisseria* and *Moraxella* spp.

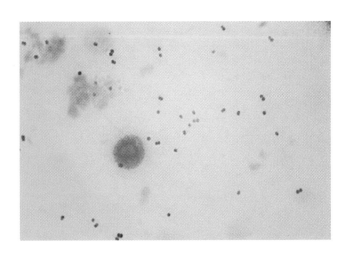

**9-1 Gram stain of *Neisseria* spp.** Gram-stained smear of a blood culture showing gram-negative diplococci characteristic of *Neisseria* spp. The adjacent sides of the cell pairs look flattened or kidney bean-shaped. The diplococci can resist decolorization and, as a result, may stain gram-variable or gram-positive (×1250).

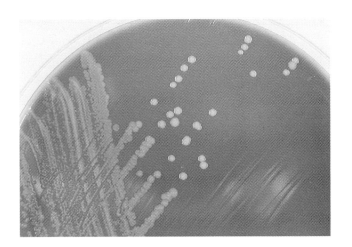

**9-2 *Neisseria meningitidis* on chocolate agar.** *Neisseria meningitidis* colonies on a chocolate agar plate incubated at 35°C in 5% $CO_2$ and 55% to 60% humidity. The colonies are more gray than yellow and nonhemolytic, characteristics that distinguish the pathogenic species of *Neisseria* from most of the nonpathogenic species. In older cultures (48 hours), a greenish cast can appear beneath the colonies in the area of heavy growth.

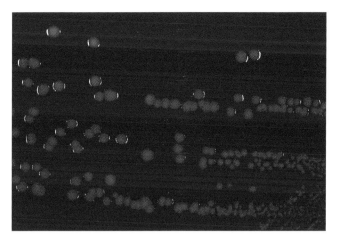

**9-3** *Neisseria meningitidis* **on 5% sheep blood agar.** Colonies are round, smooth, opaque, glistening, and 1 to 1.5 mm in diameter. The colonies are grayish in color and can appear pinkish, as shown in this figure.

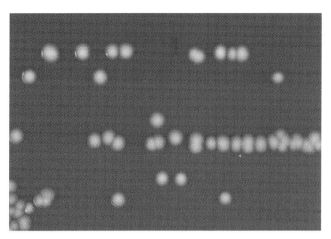

**9-4** *Neisseria gonorrhoeae* **on modified Thayer-Martin (MTM) agar.** MTM is a selective agar medium for the isolation of *N. gonorrhoeae*. It contains antimicrobial agents (vancomycin, colistin, nystatin, and trimethoprim lactate) to inhibit gram-positive and other gram-negative microorganisms, molds, some yeast, and the swarming of *Proteus* spp. After overnight incubation at 35°C in 5% $CO_2$, colonies are small (0.5 to 1.0 mm in diameter), gray, glistening, and opaque. They increase in size with prolonged incubation. Cultures should be held for 72 hours before reporting as negative.

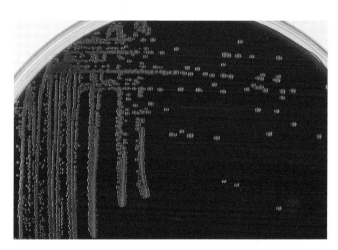

**9-5** *Moraxella (Branhamella) catarrhalis* **on 5% sheep blood agar.** *Moraxella catarrhalis* grows well on routine laboratory enriched media including blood and chocolate agar media. Colonies are usually opaque, round, and white. Microscopically, they may be confused with non-pathogenic strains of *Neisseria* spp., but they are assacharolytic in carbohydrate utilization tests, they reduce $NO_3$, and, unlike *Neisseria* spp., they produce DNase.

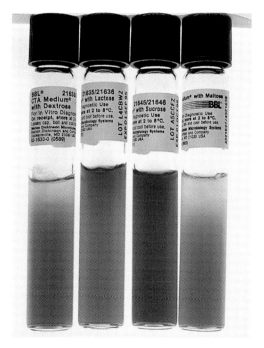

**9-6 Identification of *Neisseria* spp. by carbohydrate utilization.** The standard method for identifying *Neisseria* spp. is to determine acid in CTA (cystine-trypticase agar) medium, a semisolid agar with 1% of each of the carbohydrates glucose, lactose, maltose, and sucrose. In this example acid is produced in both glucose and maltose, identifying the isolate as *N. meningitidis*. This is an insensitive method because *Neisseria* spp. are oxidative, and the medium was designed to detect fermentative microorganisms.

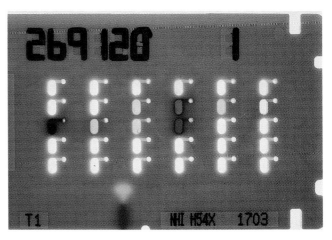

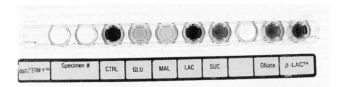

**9-7 Identification of *Neisseria* spp. by API Quad-FERM+.** API Quad-FERM+ (bioMerieux Vitek, Hazelwood, Mo.), a 2-hour method for determining carbohydrate metabolism, identifies *Neisseria* spp. and *Moraxella catarrhalis*. Tests include a carbohydrate control (CTRL), glucose (GLU), maltose (MAL), lactose (LAC) and sucrose (SUC), DNase, and beta-lactamase (b-LAC). Phenol red is the indicator. The reaction pattern shown here is characteristic of *N. meningitidis*, compared to *N. gonorrhoeae* with an acid reaction in glucose only.

**9-8 Identification of *Neisseria* spp. by *Neisseria/Haemophilus* Identification (NHI) Card.** The NHI card (bioMerieux Vitek, Hazelwood, Mo.) utilizes 16 conventional and single-substrate chromogenic tests to differentiate *Neisseria*, *Moraxella* spp., and the HACEK (*Haemophilus aphrophilus* and *H. paraphrophilus*, *Actinobacillus*, *Cardiobacterium*, *Eikenella*, and *Kingella* spp.) group of organisms. Tests include alanine-*p*-nitroanilide (ALA), phenylphosphate (OPS), proline-*p*-nitroanilide (PRO), gamma-glutamyl-*p*-nitroanilide (GGT), glycine-*p*-nitroanilide (GLY), lysine-*p*-nitroanilide (LYS), *o*-nitrophenyl-phosphorylcholine (PHC), glucose (GLU), sucrose (SUC), maltose (MLT), triphenyl-tetrazolium (TTZ), resazurin (RES), ornithine (ORN), urea (URE), and penicillin G (PEN). Indole (IND) and catalase (CAT) tests are also required. The organism in this photograph is *N. meningitidis*.

# *Haemophilus* spp.

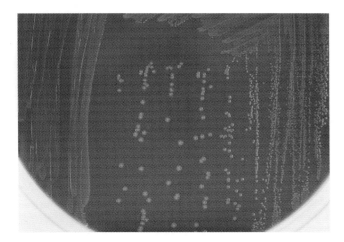

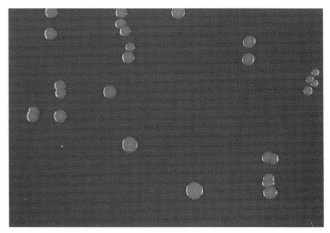

**9-9 *Haemophilus influenzae* on chocolate agar.** *Haemophilus influenzae* colonies on chocolate agar are smooth, round, entire, flat, somewhat opaque, and grayish in color. *Haemophilus influenzae* requires both X and V factors for growth; both factors are contained in chocolate agar.

**9-10 *Haemophilus influenzae* on chocolate agar (close-up view).** Colonies of mucoid, encapsulated strains of *Haemophilus influenzae* tend to be confluent, whereas nonencapsulated strains appear individually, as shown in this example. Colonies tend to have a musty odor, which has been described as smelling like "dirty sneakers."

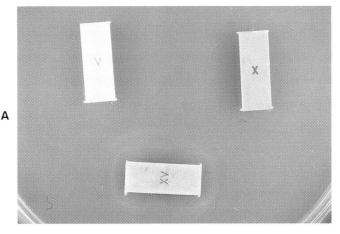

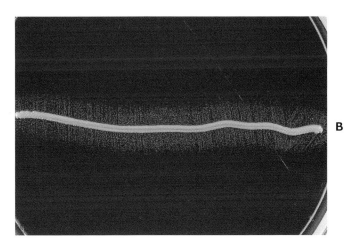

**9-11 A, Identification of *Haemophilus influenzae* by X and V strips.** The growth requirements for X-factor (heme compounds) and V-factor (nicotinamide adenine dinucleotide [NAD], also known as coenzyme I, or nicotinamide adenine dinucleotide phosphate [NADP], also known as coenzyme II) are important features for identifying *Haemophilus* spp. In this method, filter paper strips or disks are impregnated with X factor, V factor, and both factors. A suspension of organism is spread onto a medium that is devoid of the factors, and the strips are then applied. The plate is incubated overnight in 5% $CO_2$ and observed for the presence of growth surrounding the disks. This isolate grows only in the presence of both X and V factors, indicated by the faint haze of growth surrounding the XV strip. **B, *Haemophilus influenzae* satelliting around *Staphylococcus aureus*.** The blood in the agar provides the hemin (X factor), and the staphylococcus supplies the NAD (V factor), allowing growth of the *Haemophilus influenzae* near the streak.

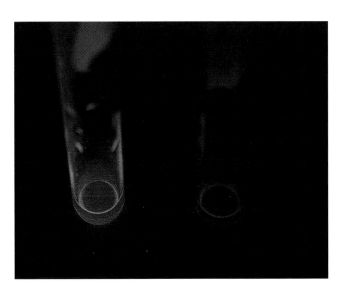

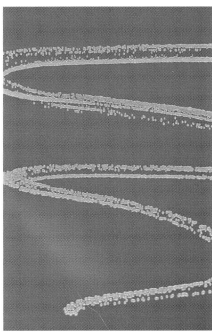

**9-12 Identification of *Haemophilus influenzae* by the Porphyrin Production Test (PPT).** This test differentiates *Haemophilus parainfluenzae* (positive) from *Haemophilus influenzae* (negative). *H. parainfluenzae* possess an enzyme, porphobilinogen synthase, that converts δ-aminolevulinic acid into porphyrins and porphobilinogen. Kovacs reagent (p-dimethylaminobenzaldehyde) detects porphobilinogen. Porphyrins produce reddish fluorescence under a Woods lamp (UV light at 360 nm). With Kovacs reagent, *H. parainfluenzae* appears red and *H. influenzae* remains colorless. Under a Woods lamp, a broth culture of *H. parainfluenzae* fluoresces and *H. influenzae* does not, as shown here.

**9-13 *Haemophilus parainfluenzae* on chocolate agar.** Colonies of *H. parainfluenzae* are approximately 3 mm in diameter, round, somewhat opaque, and glistening. This species is commonly found in the upper respiratory tract as part of the normal flora. It is important to distinguish it from *Haemophilus influenzae*, a probable pathogen in the lower respiratory tract. Both species can cause urethritis, postpartum and neonatal sepsis. Differentiation of the species is performed with the X and V strips (Figure 9-11) or the porphyrin production test (Figure 9-12).

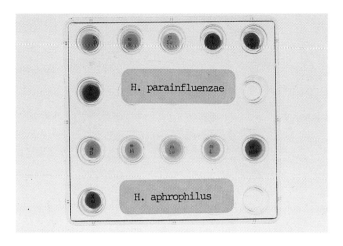

**9-14   Identification of *H. parainfluenzae* and *Haemophilus aphrophilus* with Minitek sugars.** The Minitek biochemical differentiation system (BBL Microbiology Systems, Cockeysville, Md.) utilizes paper disks impregnated with substrates to aid in the differentiation of gram-positive and gram-negative microorganisms, anaerobes, and yeast. There are approximately 40 different substrates that may be used optionally in the system. A 20-well plastic plate is used for testing. In this example, the following carbohydrates are tested: glucose (D), maltose (M), sucrose (Su), lactose (L), mannitol (MN), and xylose (X).

| | D | M | Su | L | MN | X |
|---|---|---|---|---|---|---|
| **H par** | + | + | + | 0 | 0 | 0 |
| **H aph** | + | + | + | + | 0 | 0 |

The distinguishing feature is that *Haemophilus aphrophilus* utilizes lactose.

# Bordetella, Brucella, and Pasteurella spp.

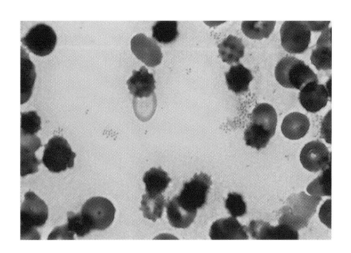

**9-15   Gram stain of *Brucella* cells (×1250).** Very tiny gram-negative bacilli isolated from a blood culture of a patient with brucellosis. Both *Bordetella* and *Pasteurella* spp. may have a similar morphology.

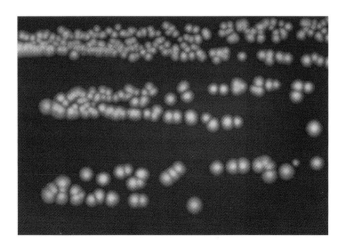

**9-16   *Bordetella bronchiseptica* on 5% sheep blood agar.** Colonies are large (3 mm in diameter), flat, and dull. They grow well on 5% sheep blood agar incubated overnight. Their appearance and odor on blood agar is similar to many of the nonfermentative gram-negative bacilli, but they do not grow on MacConkey agar. Rapid urea hydrolysis distinguishes this species from many other microorganisms.

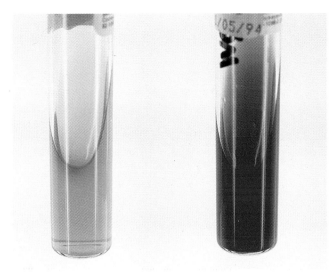

**9-17 Identification of *Bordetella bronchiseptica* by urea.** *Bordetella bronchiseptica* hydrolyzes urea rapidly. A pink color has begun to develop on the left slant 15 minutes after inoculation. The right slant turned strongly pink during overnight incubation.

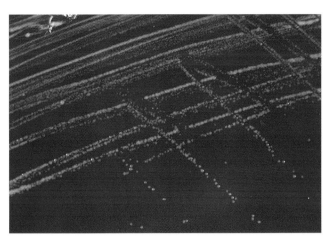

**9-18 Colonies of *Brucella* sp. on 5% sheep blood agar.** These colonies of *Brucella* are 48 hours old. These microorganisms are slow-growing, but most strains will grow on laboratory media without added enrichment. Growth may take 48 hours to become visible and even longer for a subculture from a single colony to grow. Colonies are small, raised, white to cream in color, and glistening. The agar plate should be incubated at 35°C in 5% to 10% $CO_2$ for 7 days before discarding as negative.

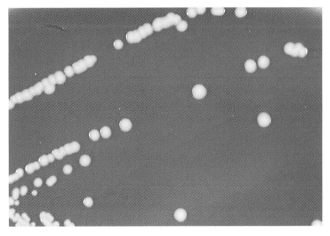

**9-19 Colonies of *Brucella* sp. on chocolate agar.** Growth of *Brucella* sp. on chocolate agar after 4 days of incubation. Colonies require prolonged incubation to attain sufficient growth for further biochemical testing.

**9-20 Identification of *Brucella* spp. by nitrate and urea.** Some *Brucella* species hydrolyze urea in less than 30 minutes and reduce nitrates to nitrites or nitrogen gas. This isolate is urease-positive and reduced $NO_3$ to $NO_2$. After 48 hours incubation in nitrate broth, sulfanilic acid and alpha-naphthylamine are added. The presence of nitrite is indicated by a red color change. If nitrate was not reduced or was reduced past nitrite to nitrogen gas, the broth remains colorless. A negative-appearing nitrate broth is confirmed by adding zinc dust, which reduces the unreduced nitrate to nitrite and causes the indicator to turn red, as shown here.

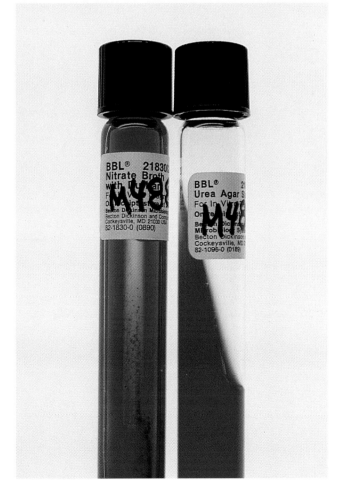

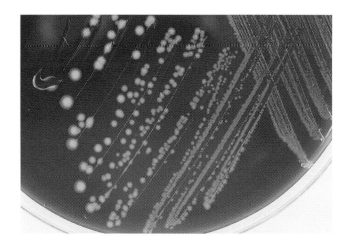

**9-21 *Pasteurella multocida* on 5% sheep blood agar.** *P. multocida* is a somewhat fastidious organism that grows slowly on 5% sheep blood agar as a round grayish, nonhemolytic colony. It is oxidase- and catalase-positive and produces indole and ornithine decarboxylase.

# *Eikenella, Kingella,* and *Capnocytophyga* spp.

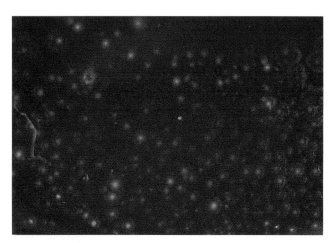

**9-22 *Eikenella corrodens* on 5% sheep blood agar.** Microscopically, *Eikenella corrodens* are tiny gram-negative bacilli. They are fastidious microorganisms and their growth is enhanced by $CO_2$ and the X factor. The microorganism grows on 5% sheep blood agar and pits or corrodes the agar surface; colony edges tend to spread. The colonies are distinguished by their bleachlike odor. The species is oxidase-positive and catalase-negative. This microorganism does not grow on MacConkey agar and is indole- and urea-negative. It does reduce nitrate to nitrite and produces lysine and ornithine decarboxylases.

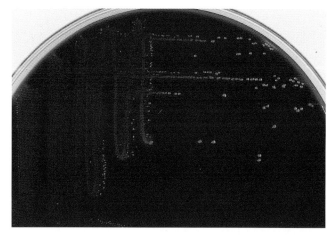

**9-23 *Kingella kingae* on 5% sheep blood agar.** Microscopically, *Kingella* spp. are plump. gram-negative coccobacilli and can appear as gram-positive because of their tendency to retain crystal violet. Colonies are oxidase-positive and catalase-negative. Colonies of *Kingella kingae* are beta-hemolytic, and the species is indole- and nitrate-negative. They are fastidious microorganisms; growth on MacConkey agar is variable.

**9-24 Colonies of *Kingella kingae* on 5% sheep blood agar showing β-hemolysis.** This figure shows the very distinct beta hemolysis displayed when the agar plate is held up to a light source.

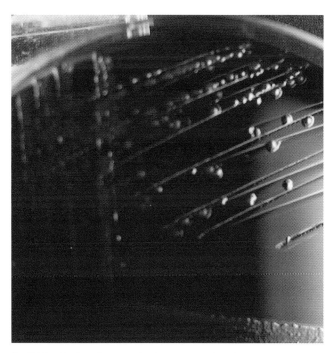

**9-25 Colonies of *Capnocytophaga* on 5% sheep blood agar.** They are fastidious, facultative anaerobes and may appear as tiny yellow colonies after overnight growth on blood agar. Growth is enhanced by $CO_2$. Colonies are slow-growing and often require 48 hours to detect distinct colonies. Microscopically, *Capnocytophaga* spp. are thin, gram-negative bacilli with pointed ends. These microorganisms were previously classified as *Bacteroides* spp. and as CDC group DF-1.

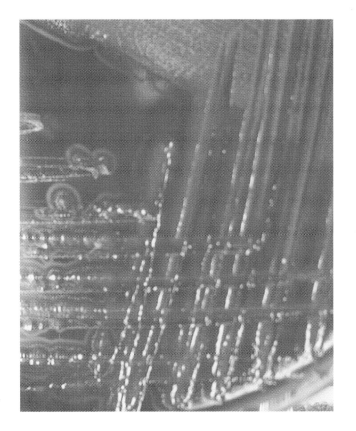

**9-26 *Capnocytophaga* on chocolate agar.** Growth on chocolate agar shows the effect of gliding motility on the colonies produced by these microorganisms. A film surrounding the colonies is characteristic for growth of this microorganism. These microorganisms do not grow on Mac-Conkey agar and are catalase-, oxidase-, indole-, and urea-negative.

# *Campylobacter* and *Vibrio* spp. (curved gram-negative bacilli)

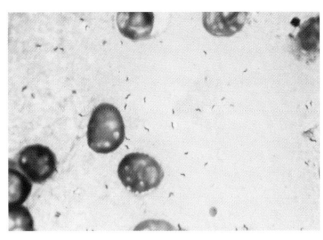

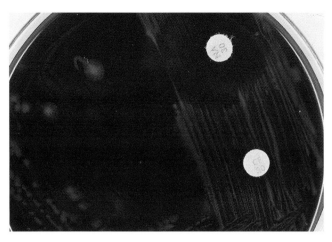

**9-27 Gram stain of *Campylobacter* spp. (×1250).** Microscopically, *Campylobacter* spp. appear as curved, comma-shaped, S-shaped, and gull-winged gram-negative bacilli. These shapes result from two cells remaining attached after division.

**9-28 Identification of *Campylobacter jejuni* by nalidixic acid susceptibility.** This microorganism grows best at 42°C, but will not grow at 25°C. It is microaerophilic, requiring 3% to 15% $O_2$ and 3% to 5% $CO_2$. Selective media (i.e., CAMPY blood agar) is required to isolate this organism from mixed flora. It is oxidase- and nitrate-positive and urea-negative. A distinguishing characteristic is its susceptibility to nalidixic acid (*top disk*) and resistance to cephalothin (*bottom disk*).

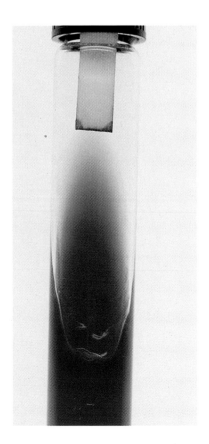

**9-29 *Campylobacter jejuni* on TSI slant with lead acetate strip.** $H_2S$ is detected with lead acetate paper, but not in the TSI medium. *Campylobacter jejuni* also hydrolyzes hippurate (Figure 6-14 on p. 40).

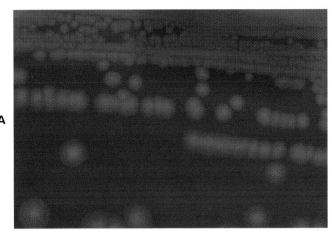

A

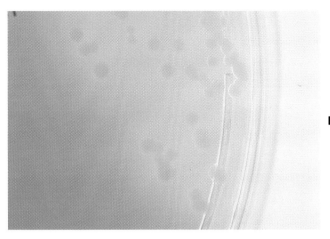

B

**9-30  A,** *Vibrio cholerae* **on 5% sheep blood agar.** Colonies of *Vibrio cholerae* grow well on most routine laboratory media. Growth is enhanced by addition of 1% NaCl. *Vibrio cholerae* tolerates 3% NaCl, is oxidase-positive, ONPG (8-12), indole-, lysine- and ornithine-positive. **B,** *Vibrio cholerae* **on thiosulfate-citrate-bile salts-sucrose (TCBS) agar.** Colonies of *Vibrio cholerae* appear yellow due to sucrose fermentation on TCBS. Most other gram-negative bacilli are inhibited.

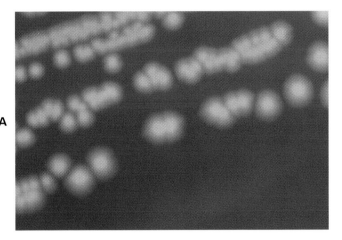

A

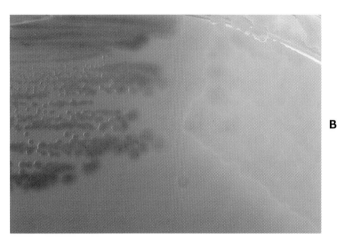

B

**9-31  A,** *Vibrio parahaemolyticus* **on 5% sheep blood agar.** *Vibrio parahaemolyticus* does require NaCl for growth and can tolerate 8% NaCl. Colonies on 5% sheep blood agar are approximately 1 to 3 mm in diameter, dull, and can assume a pale blue-green color. Colonies grow well on MacConkey agar, are indole-, oxidase-, lysine-, and ornithine decarboxylase-positive. This species ferments glucose, maltose, and mannitol. This organism has been associated with wound infections and gastroenteritis. **B,** *Vibrio parahaemolyticus* **(green colonies) and** *V. cholerae* **(yellow colonies) on TCBS.** *V. parahaemolyticus* does not ferment sucrose; thus colonies are green.

# Nonfermentative Gram-Negative Bacilli

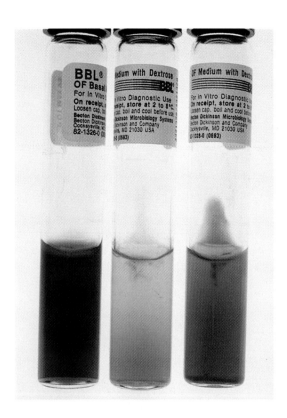

**9-32 Oxidative-fermentative (OF) medium.** Bacteria incorporate carbohydrates by both oxidative and fermentative pathways, as detected in OF medium (Hugh and Leifson's) with bromthymol blue pH indicator. The low protein-to-carbohydrate ratio in OF media prevents the neutralization of weak acid by alkaline end-products. The microorganisms described in this section are oxidative and nonoxidative gram-negative bacilli. The tube on the left contains the basal medium alone; the other two tubes contain dextrose. A positive test (oxidative) is indicated by a yellow color (*center tube*) and a negative test (nonoxidative, nonfermentative) shows no color change (*green, right tube*). Fermentative microorganisms produce acid in both the oxidative (open) tube and the fermentative tube (overlaid with mineral oil, Figure 5-6 on p. 33).

## *Pseudomonadaceae*

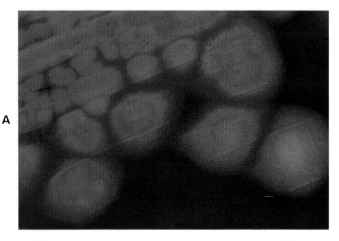

A

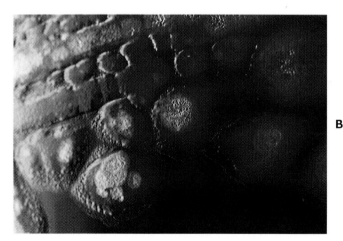

B

**9-33 A,** *Pseudomonas aeruginosa* **on 5% sheep blood agar.** The colonies of *P. aeruginosa* on blood agar are typically yellow-green and beta-hemolytic. Fluorescein pigments are produced by some species, but pyocyanin (blue-green) pigment is produced by *P. aeruginosa* alone. Most colonies have a distinct grapelike odor due to aminoacetophenone. *P. aeruginosa* may be distinguished from other species by its ability to grow at 42°C. **B,** *Pseudomonas aeruginosa* **on 5% sheep blood agar.** Oblique lighting demonstrates metallic sheen on the surface of colonies.

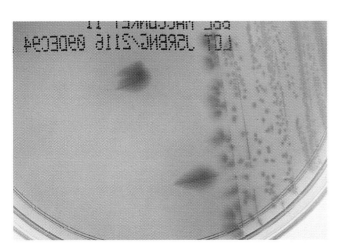

**9-34** *Pseudomonas aeruginosa* **on Mac-Conkey agar.** Flat, blue-green colonies with very distinct feathered edges growing on MacConkey agar. Colonies grow well at 35°C aerobically. They will also grow at 25°C.

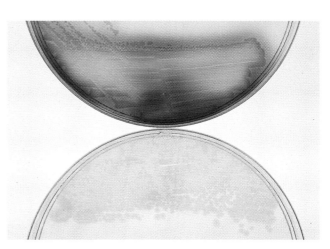

**9-35 Pigment production by** *Pseudomonas aeruginosa.* Two strains of *Pseudomonas aeruginosa* growing on MacConkey agar. The red pigment is due to the production of pyorubrin, a nonfluorescent, water-soluble pigment, and the yellow-green color is due to pyocyanin, a fluorescent, water-soluble pigment.

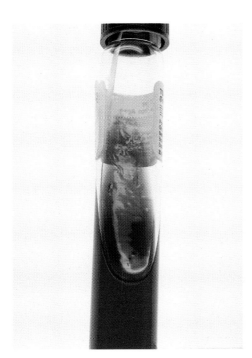

**9-36** *Pseudomonas aeruginosa* **on TSI slant.** On a TSI agar slant *Pseudomonas aeruginosa* appears as a blue-green, somewhat metallic, fluorescent layer of growth.

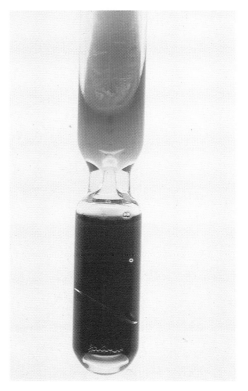

**9-37 Identification of** *Pseudomonas aeruginosa* **by characteristics in GNF tube.** The N/F System (Remel Laboratories, Lenexa, Kan.) is used for the identification of gram-negative bacilli that do not belong to the *Enterobacteriaceae.* The system consists of the GNF (glucose-$N_2$-fluorescein) tube, the 42P tube (Figure 9-38) and the Uni-N/F-Tek plate (Figure 9-39). This microorganism produces a fluorescing pigment (under a Woods lamp). The red area under the constriction indicates $N_2$ gas production. *P. aeruginosa* does not ferment glucose.

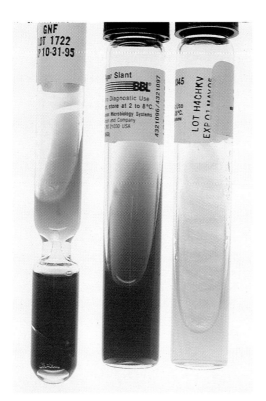

**9-38 Identification of *Pseudomonas aerugi-nosa* by GNF, urea, and Pseudosel (42P) agar.** In this figure the GNF slant described in Figure 9-37 is on the left, a positive urea slant (Figure 8-16 on p. 61) is in the center, and 42P, the second tube of the N/F screen, is on the right. The 42P medium, also known as pseudosel agar, is incubated at 42°C for 18 to 24 hours. This microorganism grew at 42°C and produced the blue-green pyocyanin pigment. Based on the reactions in this figure, the microorganism can be definitively identified as *Pseudomonas aeruginosa*.

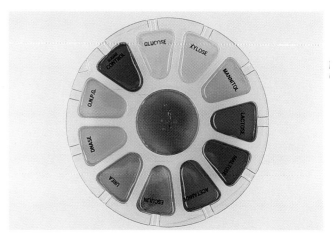

**9-39 Identification of *Pseudomonas aerugi-nosa* by Uni-N/F-Tek Plate.** The Uni-N/F-Tek plate (Remel Laboratories, Lenexa, Kan.) is a 13 test unit consisting of H$_2$S, indole, a carbohydrate control, glucose, xylose, mannitol, lactose, maltose, acetamide, esculin, urea, DNase, and ONPG (Figure 8-12 on p. 59). Reactions for *Pseudomonas aeruginosa* are:

| GLU | XYL | MAN | LAC | MAL | ACET |
|---|---|---|---|---|---|
| + | + | + | + | 0 | 0 |
| **ESC** | **Urea** | **DNase** | **ONPG** | **H$_2$S** | **IND** |
| 0 | + | + | + | 0 | 0 |

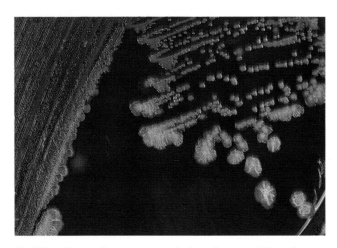

**9-40 *Pseudomonas stutzeri* on 5% sheep blood agar.** Characteristic colonies of *Pseudomonas stutzeri* on 5% sheep blood agar are buff-colored, dry, wrinkled, and adhere to the agar surface, making it difficult to remove them from the plate. Most strains grow at 42°C and reduce nitrates to nitrogen gas.

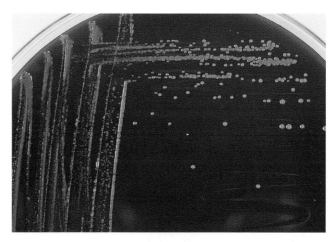

**9-41 *Sphingomonas* (formerly *Pseudomonas*) *paucimobilis* on 5% sheep blood agar.** Colonies of *Sphingomonas paucimobilis* on 5% sheep blood agar are small and yellow-pigmented after 24 hours of incubation. This species was previously known as *Pseudomonas paucimobilis* and CDC group llk-1. It is a slow-growing microorganism at 35°C, but optimal growth occurs at 30°C. This microorganism does not grow at 42°C or on MacConkey agar. It is oxidase-, esculin-, ONPG-, and DNase-positive and nitrate- and indole-negative.

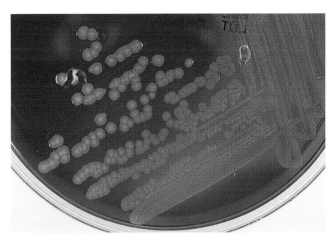

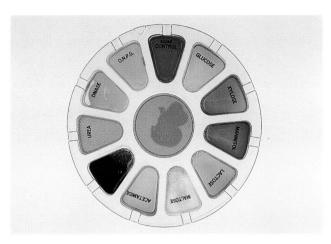

**9-42** *Stenotrophomonas (Xanthomonas) maltophilia* **on 5% sheep blood agar.** Colonies of *Stenotrophomonas maltophilia* on 5% sheep blood agar are chartreuse to lavender-green and have a characteristic strong ammonia odor. Unlike other pseudomonads, this species is oxidase-negative. It is resistant to many antimicrobials, although trimethoprim-sulfamethoxazole is usually effective.

**9-43 Identification of *Stenotrophomonas (Xanthomonas) maltophilia* by the Uni-N/F-Tek.** Reactions for *Stenotrophomonas maltophilia* are:

| GLU | XYL | MAN | LAC | MAL | ACET |
|---|---|---|---|---|---|
| weak | 0 | 0 | 0 | + | 0 |
| **ESC** | **Urea** | **DNase** | **ONPG** | **H$_2$S** | **IND** |
| + | + | + | + | 0 | 0 |

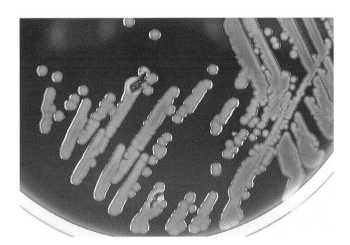

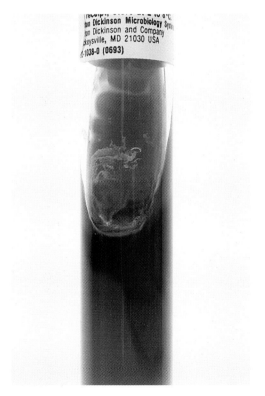

**9-44** *Shewanella (Pseudomonas) putrefaciens* **on 5% sheep blood agar.** *Shewanella* is the new genus name for the microorganism previously classified as *Pseudomonas putrefaciens* and CDC group lb. Colonies of *Shewanella putrefaciens* on 5% sheep blood agar are slightly viscous and mucoid and pinkish to red-brown or orange-tan in color.

**9-45 TSI reaction of *Shewanella (Pseudomonas) putrefaciens*.** The key characteristic that differentiates *Pseudomonas putrefaciens* from frequently encountered nonfermenters and other related microorganisms is its ability to produce large amounts of H$_2$S in TSI or KIA slants.

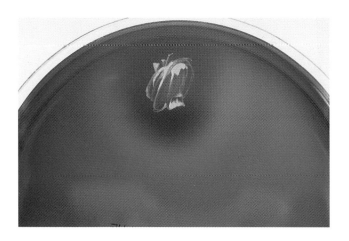

**9-46 DNase agar.** Production of the enzyme DNase, which hydrolyzes DNA, may be used to differentiate nonfermenting gram-negative bacteria as well as *Staphylococcus aureus* and *Serratia marcescens.* This DNase test medium contains toluidine blue complexed with DNA. Hydrolysis of DNA by the inoculated microorganism causes changes of structure of the dye to yield a pink color. Toluidine blue may inhibit growth of some microorganisms, so equivocal results should be retested with another method.

# Other Nonfermentative Bacilli

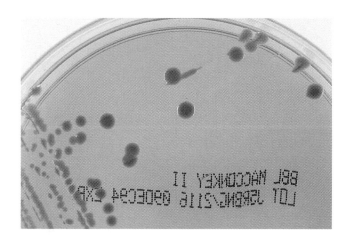

**9-47 *Acinetobacter (Acinetobacter calcoaceticus var. anitratus) baumannii* on Mac-Conkey agar.** *Acinetobacter baumannii* was formerly designated as *Acinetobacter calcoaceticus* var. *anitratus, Moraxella lwoffi, Herellea vaginicola,* and *Mima polymorpha.* They do not produce a pigment on blood agar, but appear faint pink on MacConkey agar, as shown in this figure. They are oxidase- and nitrate-negative. Microscopically, these microorganisms appear as coccobacilli, predominantly in pairs, and for this reason they have been confused with *Neisseria* and *Moraxella* spp.

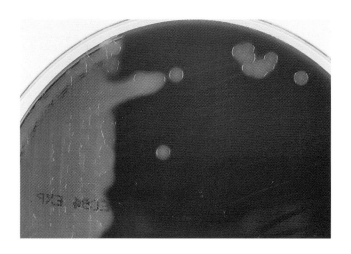

**9-48 *Flavobacterium meningosepticum* on 5% sheep blood agar.** Colonies of *Flavobacterium meningosepticum* on 5% sheep blood agar after 48 hours of incubation are approximately 3 mm in diameter. Growth on MacConkey agar is variable, and most strains are oxidase-positive. This species is indole-, esculin-, ONPG-, and DNase-positive, urea-negative, and nonmotile.

**9-49** *Burkholderia (Pseudomonas) cepacia on MacConkey agar.* This species, formerly known as *Pseudomonas cepacia,* grows slowly, especially when recovered from cystic fibrosis patients, in whom it is a significant pathogen. Colonies on MacConkey agar are often bright pink or red after prolonged incubation (as shown here) due to lactose oxidation. The species is oxidase-positive, although many strains display a weak oxidase reactivity. Most strains are lysine decarboxylase-positive and oxidize a number of sugars, including lactose.

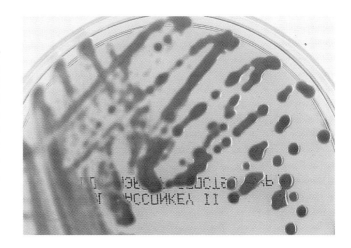

**9-50** *Legionella pneumophila* on **buffered charcoal-yeast extract (BCYE) agar.** BCYE agar is a selective medium for the recovery of *Legionella* spp. This buffered medium is the agar of choice for the isolation of *Legionella* spp. because it contains the requirements for optimal growth of the microorganism; L-cysteine, iron salts, and a pH of 6.9. Antibiotics are added to inhibit the growth of other bacteria. Growth appears in 2 to 3 days, and the colonies are circular, glistening, entire, and measure up to 4 mm, as shown here.

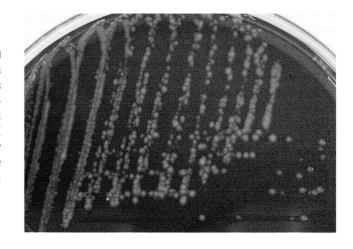

# CHAPTER 10 *Anaerobic Bacteria*

**A**naerobic bacteria are unable to multiply in the presence of atmospheric oxygen, although they have varying degrees of oxygen tolerance. The pathogenic strains are divided into two groups: exogenous pathogens, primarily the spore-forming clostridia that live in the soil and contaminate wounds or sporulate in foods to cause disease; and the endogenous pathogens, normal inhabitants of human mucosa or lumens that cause disease when they enter a normally sterile site after traumatic breakdown of the normal mucosal integrity.

Specimens must be protected from air during collection, transport, and laboratory handling to maximize recovery of these fastidious microorganisms. Because of the time and resources necessary to perform good anaerobic microbiology, most laboratories limit anaerobic processing to specimens likely to harbor anaerobes, such as abscess aspirates, deep tissue biopsies, and specimens collected through a protected catheter system.

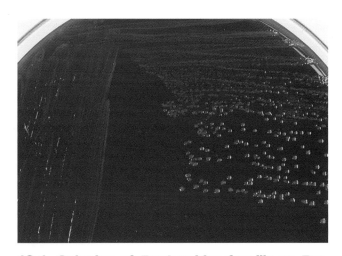

**10-1 Colonies of *Bacteroides fragilis* on *Brucella* blood agar.** *Bacteroides* spp. as well as other anaerobic gram-negative bacilli grow best on this nonselective medium. Agar must be supplemented with hemin and vitamin K1 to support the growth of many species of anaerobes. These colonies appear as circular, entire, and raised.

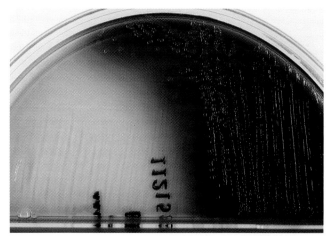

**10-2 Colonies of *Bacteroides fragilis* on *Bacteroides* bile esculin (BBE) agar.** This medium contains gentamicin to inhibit facultative gram-negative bacilli. Bile salts inhibit most anaerobes other than those of the *B. fragilis* group, which grow as large, gray to black colonies due to their hydrolysis of esculin in the medium.

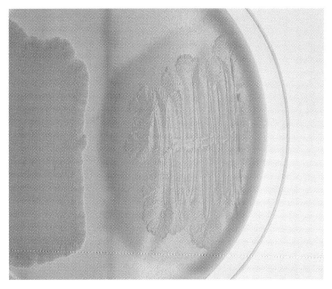

**10-3 Growth of clostridia on egg yolk agar.**
The production of the enzymes lecithinase, opaque white precipitate extending from the colony into the medium (*right side*), and lipase, iridescent sheen on surface of colony (*left side*) is used to differentiate among *Clostridium* species and to help identify some *Fusobacterium* species.

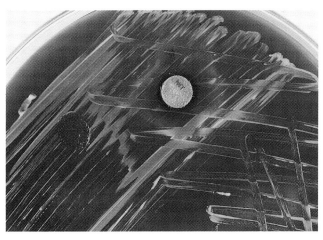

**10-4 Nitrate disk test.** To test for reduction of nitrate to nitrite, a nitrate-impregnated filter paper disk is placed onto the inoculum of an anaerobic subculture of the microorganism. After 48 hours incubation, drops of the nitrate reagents, sulfanilic acid and alpha-naphthylamine, are added to the disk. A red color indicates the presence of nitrite.

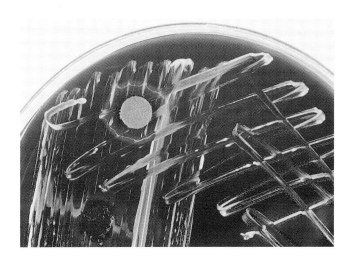

**10-5 Spot indole disk test.** To test for presence of the enzyme tryptophanase, a plain filter paper disk is placed on an area of growth of a microorganism on a medium containing tryptophan (such as most blood agar bases). After the disk has become moist (5 minutes), a drop of paradimethylaminocinnamaldehyde is placed on the disk. A greenish-blue color indicates the presence of indole, a breakdown product of tryptophan. Indole is used to help differentiate among some *Fusobacterium, Propionibacterium, Porphyromonas, Prevotella,* and *Peptostreptococcus* spp.

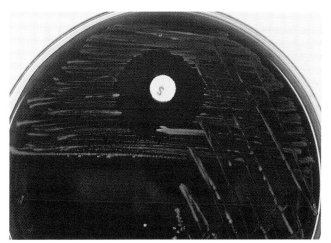

**10-6 Sodium polyanethol sulfonate (SPS) disk test.** *Peptostreptococcus anaerobius* is the only anaerobic gram-positive coccus that is inhibited by SPS.

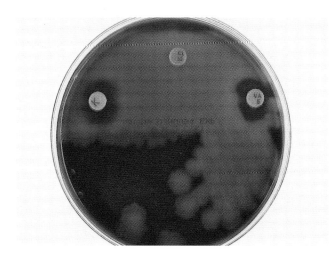

**10-7  Special potency antimicrobial disks for presumptive identification of anaerobes.** The pattern of susceptibility to the three antibiotic disks: kanamycin (1000 μg), colistin (10 μg), and vancomycin (5 μg) can help differentiate among anaerobic genera using these criteria:

| Microorganism type | Kanamycin | Vancomycin | Colistin |
|---|---|---|---|
| *Clostridium* | S (1, 2) | S | R |
| *Bacteroides fragilis* group | R (1) | R | R |
| *Bacteroides ureolyticus* group | S | R | S |
| *Fusobacterium* species | S | R | S |
| *Veillonella* species | S | R | S |
| *Porphyromonas* species | R | S | R |
| *Prevotella* species | R | R | V |
| *Peptostreptococcus anaerobius* | R (3) | S | R |
| Other gram-positive cocci | S | S | R |

(1)  Some strains are kanomycin-resistant
(2)  V, variable; R, resistant; S, susceptible
(3)  Rare strains are susceptible

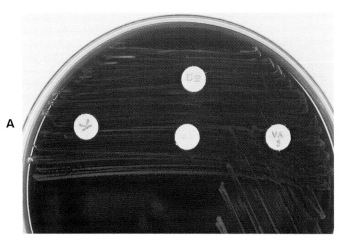

A

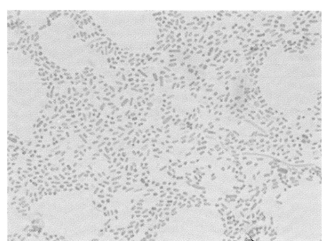

B

**10-8  A,** *Bacteroides fragilis* **on Brucella blood agar.** The large gray, mucoid colonies and resistance to all three potency disks described in Figure 10-7 are typical of members of the *B. fragilis* group. The extra filter paper disk is for performance of the nitrate test. **B, Gram stain of** *Bacteroides fragilis.* Pale-staining, gram-negative bacilli with rounded ends. Both pleomorphism and irregularity in staining can be observed in this smear (×1250).

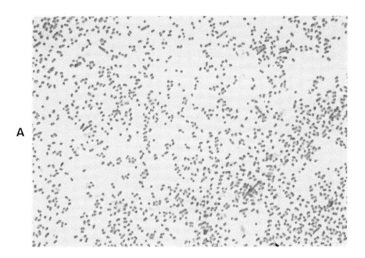

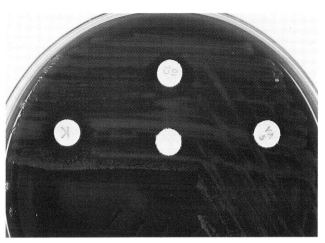

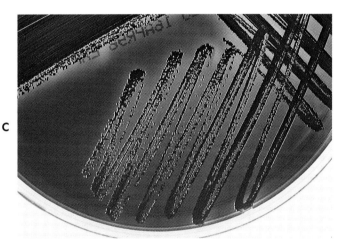

**10-9 A, Gram stain of *Prevotella melanino-genica* (×1250).** Small, pleomorphic, gram-negative coc cobacilli and bacilli can be observed in this smear, a character-istic appearance of *Prevotella melaninogenica*. **B, *Prevotella melaninogenica* on *Brucella* blood agar.** The small, dark-appearing colonies, resistant to kanamycin (less than 10 mm zone of inhibition) and vancomycin, will fluo-resce brick-red under ultraviolet light (Woods lamp). **C, *Prevotella melaninogenica* on *Brucella* blood agar.** After several more days of incubation, these colonies will take on a dark brown to black color, due to assimilation of heme in the medium.

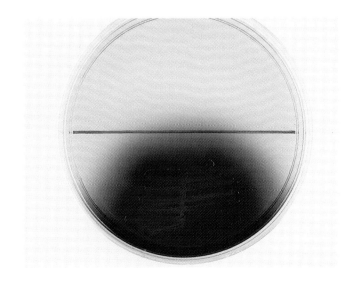

**10-10 *Bacteroides fragilis* and *Prevotella melaninogenica* on *Bacteroides* bile esculin (BBE) agar.** The *Prevotella* species was streaked on the up-per half of the plate, but growth was inhibited. The *Bacteroides fragilis* grows profusely, displaying a typical gray precipitate in the agar surrounding the colonies.

A

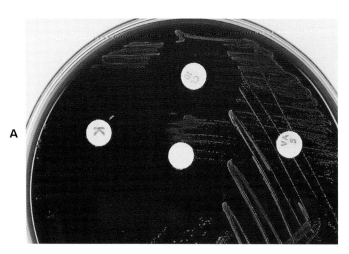

B

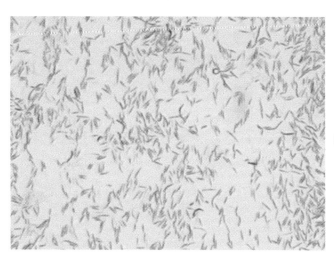

**10-11  A, *Fusobacterium nucleatum* on *Brucella* blood agar.** The dry, white, breadcrumblike colonies (one colony variant of this species) and the antibiotic disk pattern (kanamycin- and colistin-susceptible; vancomycin-resistant) are suggestive of *F. nucleatum.* If indole reagent is added to the extra filter paper disk on the plate, the disk will turn blue because this species is indole-positive. **B, Gram stain of *Fusobacterium nucleatum* (×1250).** Pale-staining, long, slender, gram-negative bacilli with tapered/pointed ends demonstrating the characteristic appearance of *Fusobacterium nucleatum.*

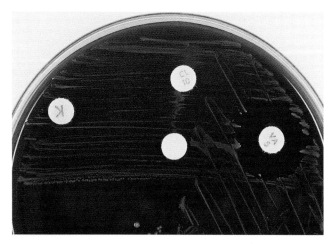

**10-12  *Peptostreptococcus anaerobius* on *Brucella* blood agar.** This gram-negative coccus displays medium-sized gray colonies, resistance to kanamycin and colistin, and susceptibility to vancomycin.

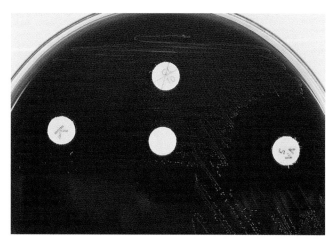

**10-13  *Peptostreptococcus magnus* on *Brucella* blood agar.** This species has tiny colonies but Gram stain yields large, micrococcus-appearing gram-positive cocci. It is susceptible to kanamycin and vancomycin and resistant to colistin.

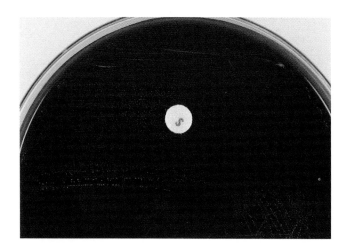

**10-14  Sodium polyanetholsulfonate (SPS) resistance of *Peptostreptococcus magnus.*** Unlike *P. anaerobius, P. magnus* is resistant to SPS.

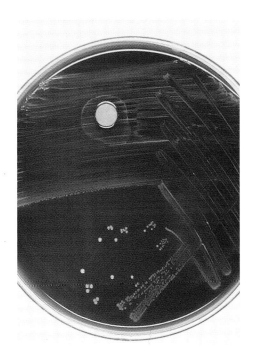

**10-15 Colonies of *Proprionibacterium acnes* on *Brucella* blood agar.** These young colonies are small and white to gray-white; however, as they age, they can appear yellowish. They have been referred to as anaerobic diphtheroids because, when stained and examined microscopically, they resemble diphtheroids. *Proprionibacterium acnes* are indol-positive, as seen on this plate, and catalase-positive. When an anaerobic diphtheroid is catalase- and indol-positive, it can be presumptively identified as *Proprionibacterium acnes*.

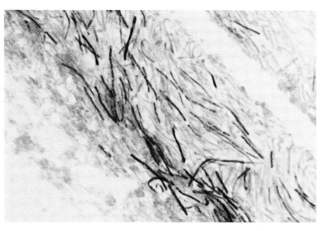

**10-16 Gram stain of *Clostridium* species (×1250).** Cells are parallel-sided, long, thin, gram-variable, and some show swollen ends indicative of spore formation.

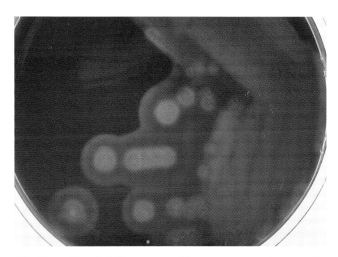

**10-17 *Clostridium perfringens* on *Brucella* blood agar.** Colonies display the double-zone of beta hemolysis typical of this species. Colonies are large with peaked centers and irregular edges after 48 hours incubation.

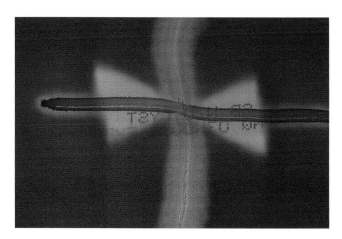

**10-18 Reverse CAMP test for presumptive identification of *Clostridium perfringens*.** *C. perfringens* is streaked vertically, and *Streptococcus agalactiae* is streaked horizontally in this test. The hemolysis of the clostridium is synergistically enhanced by the hemolysin of the streptococcus in an arrowhead-shaped pattern.

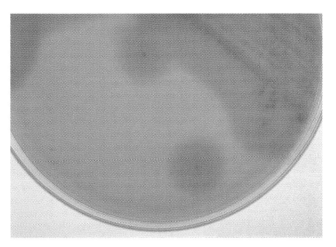

**10-19 *Clostridium perfringens* on egg yolk agar.** Colonies and surrounding medium display the expanding white precipitate stimulated by lecithinase production, typical of *C. perfringens*.

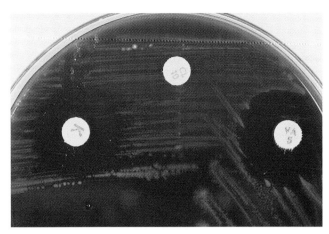

**10-20   *Clostridium difficile* on *Brucella* blood agar.** Colonies show the special potency disk pattern indicative of a gram-positive microorganism. This species has a distinctive barnyard odor and will fluoresce chartreuse under ultraviolet light. Laboratory diagnosis of *Clostridium difficile* diarrhea usually depends on detection of the toxin in feces, rather than on isolation of the microorganism.

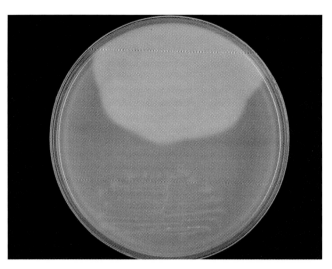

**10-21   *Clostridium difficile* and *C. perfringens* on egg yolk agar.** The *C. perfringens* (*upper half of plate*) produces abundant lecithinase, while the *C. difficile* (*lower half*) grows but shows no reaction.

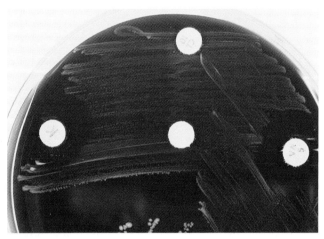

**10-22   *Clostridium tertium* on *Brucella* blood agar.** This species also shows the special potency disk pattern indicative of a gram-positive organism. *C. tertium* is one of several species of *Clostridium* that is able to grow aerobically. Spores are formed more readily, however, during anaerobic growth.

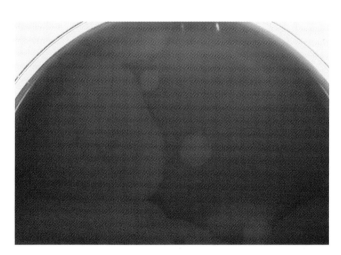

**10-23   *Clostridium tetani* on *Brucella* blood agar.** Growth on agar is characterized by swarming, such that growth will cover the entire plate in a thin film within a few days.

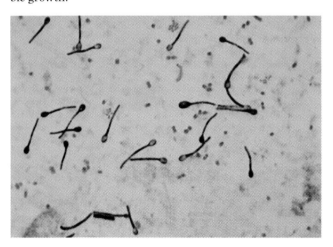

**10-24   Gram stain of *Clostridium paraputrificum* (×1250).** This microorganism displays terminal, swollen spores and the gram-variable staining typical of *Clostridium* species. Spores may not take up the stain, so they may appear as clear areas.

# CHAPTER 11 *Mycobacteria*

T he *Mycobacterium* species include the *Mycobacterium tuberculosis* complex and the nontuberculous mycobacteria. They are slender, rod-shaped aerobic bacteria that require special media for growth. Acid-fastness is a key characteristic of these bacteria. Mycobacteria may be divided into slow and rapid growers. Slow growers require at least 7 days of incubation to produce visible colonies, while colonies of rapid growers usually appear in less than 7 days. The rapid growers may be confused with other related genera, *Corynebacterium*, *Nocardia*, and *Rhodococcus*, because they may be partially acid-fast.

**11-1 Kinyoun's acid fast stain (×1500).** Mycobacteria are readily stained with carbol fuchsin, which binds the mycolic acid in their lipid-rich cell walls. This stain cannot be removed (decolorized) with acid alcohol and, therefore, the microorganisms are referred to as acid-fast. There are two common acid-fast stains, Ziehl-Neelsen (ZN), and Kinyoun's. The difference is that the ZN stain requires heat during the staining process because the phenol concentration used is less than in the Kinyoun's method. The decolorizer, acid alcohol, and the counterstain, methylene blue, are the same for both methods. When stained, acid-fast bacilli stain red and the background is blue, as shown here.

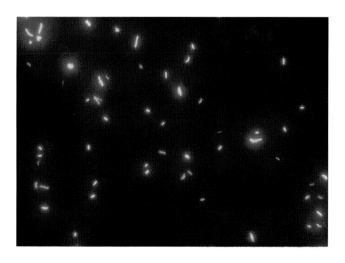

**11-2 Auramine fluorescent stain (×1250).** In this method, a fluorescent dye is used to bind the mycolic acid in the cell walls of mycobacteria. Both auramine and rhodamine are fluorochromes that can be used to stain mycobacteria. When stained with a fluorochrome, mycobacteria are bright yellow (auramine O), as shown here, or orange-red (rhodamine), with a black background due to the potassium permanganate counterstain. The advantage of the fluorochrome stain is that the slides can be scanned using a ×25 objective, instead of the ×100 oil-immersion objective that is required to examine carbol fuchsin–stained smears. This lower magnification increases the viewing field and decreases the reading time.

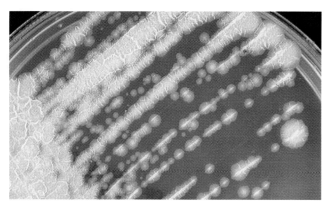

**11-3** *M. tuberculosis* **on Middlebrook 7H11 agar.** Colonies appear as cream-colored, dry, and wrinkled. Middlebrook 7H11 agar is a widely used medium for the isolation and antimicrobial susceptibility testing of mycobacteria. Although similar to Middlebrook 7H10 agar, 7H11 agar contains casein hydrolysates that improve the recovery of isoniazid-resistant strains of *M. tuberculosis* and shortens the incubation time for *M. avium* complex isolates. Seen here is a rough colony of *M. tuberculosis* growing on Middlebrook 7H11 agar.

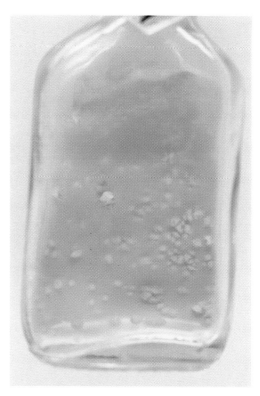

**11-4** *M. tuberculosis* **on Löwenstein-Jensen (LJ) agar slant.** LJ agar has been used as the standard for isolating mycobacteria. It contains coagulated whole eggs, glycerol, potato flour, and salts. Malachite green is added to inhibit the growth of contaminating bacteria. The disadvantage of this medium is that it becomes hydrolyzed when contaminants do grow on it, and the culture must be discarded. Illustrated here are rough, buff-colored colonies that appeared within 3 weeks, typical of *M. tuberculosis*.

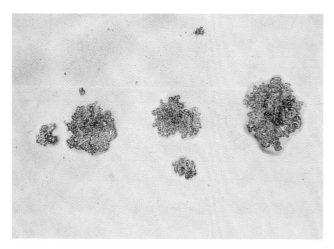

**11-5 Colonies of** *M. tuberculosis* **(×10).** Very young colonies (less than 10 days old) growing on Middlebrook 7H11 agar. Viewed microscopically, the very beginning of the cording characteristic of *M. tuberculosis* can be observed.

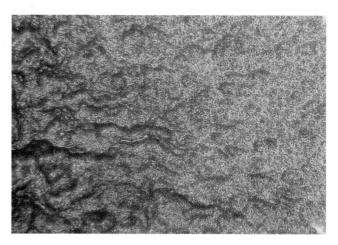

**11-6 Colonies of** *M. tuberculosis* **(×75).** Older colonies (3 to 4 weeks old) growing on Middlebrook 7H11 agar. The colonies have a rough appearance and exhibit cording, exemplified by the darker areas.

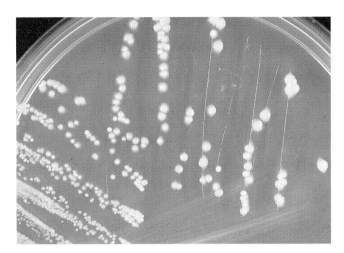

**11-7 *M. avium* on Middlebrook 7H11 agar.** Two distinct colony types of *M. avium* are shown on this Middlebrook 7H11 agar plate; a smaller, smooth colony that is slightly opaque and a larger, rough colony. Pure cultures containing both colony types are characteristic of *M. avium*. In most cases, *M. avium* strains can be distinguished from other *M. avium*-complex microorganisms, such as *M. intracellulare*, by their ability to grow at 45°C.

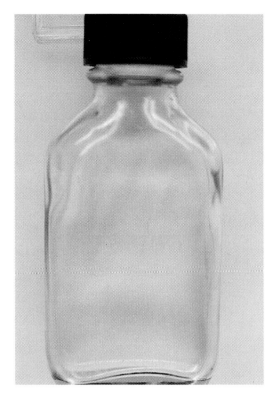

**11-8 *M. avium* on Löwenstein-Jensen agar slant.** *M. avium* does not grow well on LJ agar. It appears as a film after 3 to 4 weeks of incubation. Colonies are buff-colored as shown here, but much smaller than *M. tuberculosis* (compare with Figure 11-4).

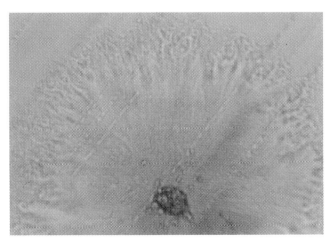

**11-9 Smooth colony of *M. avium* (×15).** Microscopically, the smooth colony type can appear as a "sun-spot" with starlike or asteroid margins as shown here.

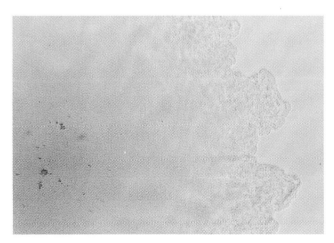

**11-10 Rough colony of *M. avium* (×15).** This view of the rough colony has a characteristic "lacy" appearance.

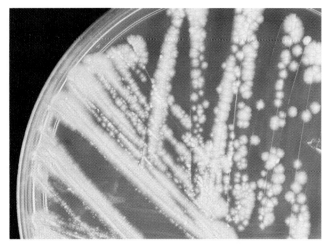

**11-11  *M. kansasii* on Middlebrook 7H11 agar.**
*M. kansasii* is a photochromogen, group I of Runyon's classification, a classical method for differentiating the mycobacteria. Growth appears on Middlebrook 7H11 agar in approximately 3 weeks. A characteristic feature of the photochromogens is their dependence on exposure to light for pigment production. Shown here are the rough, wrinkled colonies of *M. kansasii* before exposure to light. The colonies are buff-colored.

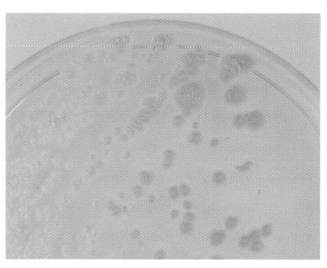

**11-12  *M. kansasii* on Middlebrook 7H11 agar.**
Following exposure to light for a few hours, colonies of *M. kansasii* have a strong yellow color. Further characteristics of *M. kansasii* include a positive catalase reaction, reduction of nitrate to nitrite, and rapid hydrolysis of Tween 80, a detergent.

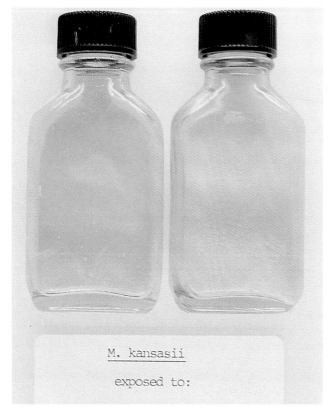

**11-13  *M. kansasii* on Löwenstein-Jensen agar.**
The slant on the left was exposed to light, resulting in the strong yellow-colored colonies, while the slant on the right was not exposed to light and the colonies remained buff-colored.

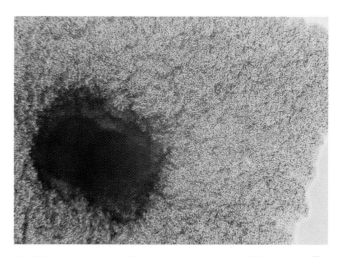

**11-14  Colony of *M. kansasii* (×75).** Microscopically, this 3-week-old colony growing on Middlebrook 7H11 agar shows a dark, dense center and a wrinkled periphery, a characteristic of *M. kansasii.*

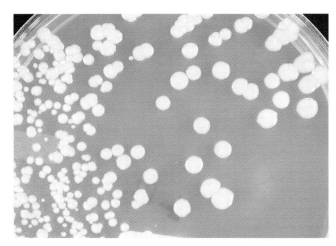

**11-15** *M. chelonae* **on Middlebrook 7H11 agar.** This rapid grower can appear on culture media within 2 to 4 days. *M. chelonae* belongs to the *M. fortuitum-chelonae* complex. *M. chelonae* can be distinguished from *M. fortuitum* because it does not reduce nitrates or assimilate iron, but it is susceptible to polymyxin B and resistant to ciprofloxacin.

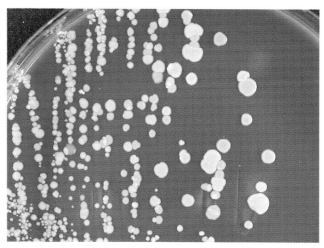

**11-16** *M. chelonae* **on chocolate agar.** *M. chelonae* can grow on chocolate agar and appear as smooth, opaque colonies resembling staphylococci or yeast. Because these microorganisms can be associated with skin infections and can be confused morphologically with other isolates also associated with skin infections, definitive identification of such colonies is needed. Although they are not readily stained by the Gram stain, they may appear as weakly staining, beaded, gram-positive bacilli, suggesting the possibility of a rapidly growing mycobacterium.

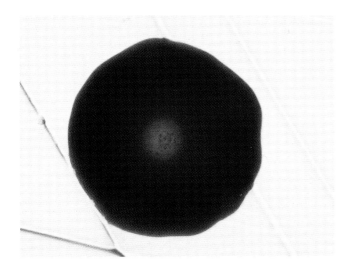

**11-17 Colony of** *M. chelonae* **(×20).** Examined microscopically, the colonies appear dark and dense with smooth edges and a somewhat lighter center, as shown here.

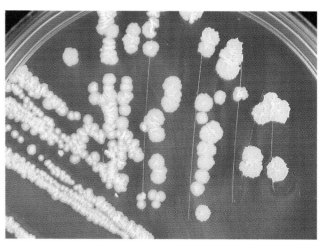

**11-18** *M. fortuitum* **on Middlebrook 7H11 agar.** The rapidly growing, rough colonies are shown after 3 days of incubation. *M. fortuitum* can also grow on modified MacConkey agar, without crystal violet, at 37°C, at 43°C on 7H11 and LJ, and in 5% NaCl at 37°C. These characteristics help to distinguish this species from *M. chelonae.*

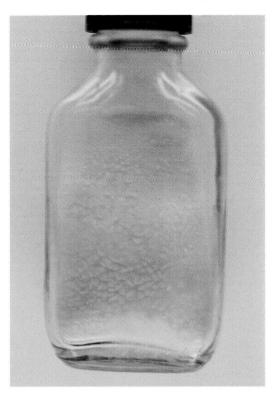

**11-19** *M. fortuitum* **on Löwenstein-Jensen agar.** The rough colonies are shown growing on LJ agar after 3 days of incubation.

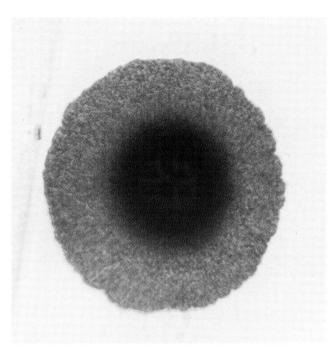

**11-20 Colony of** *M. fortuitum* **(×20).** The rough colony of *M. fortuitum* observed microscopically with transmitted light demonstrates a somewhat smooth edge with a very dense center.

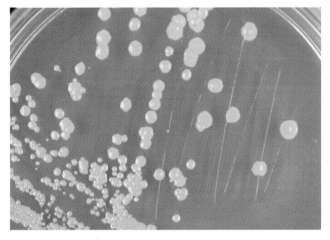

**11-21** *M. gordonae* **on Middlebrook 7H11 agar.** Yellow-orange pigmented colonies of *M. gordonae*. This species belong to the Runyon group II scotochromogens, characterized by pigmented colonies in the absence of exposure to light. Colony growth can appear in 3 weeks.

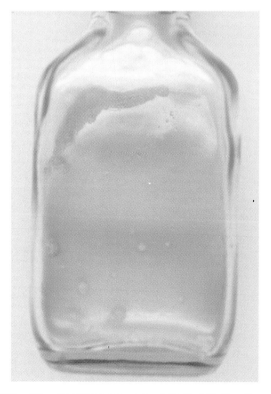

**11-22** *M. gordonae* **on Löwenstein-Jensen agar.** The yellow-orange pigment is also produced on LJ agar.

**11-23 Colony of *M. gordonae* on Middlebrook 7H11 agar (×15).** The entire colony is dense and dark when examined microscopically with transmitted light.

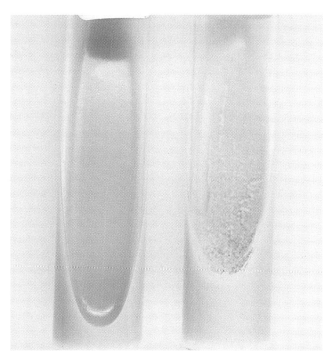

**11-24 Sodium chloride tolerance test.** Some species of mycobacteria, including the rapid growers except for *M. chelonae*, can grow at 28°C on an egg-based medium containing 5% NaCl. *M. chelonae* does not grow (*left*), while *M. fortuitum* grows (*right*).

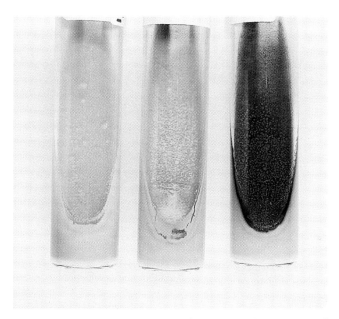

**11-25 Iron uptake test.** The iron uptake test is used mainly to differentiate *M. fortuitum* and other rapid growers from *M. chelonae*. *M. fortuitum* and other rapid growers have the ability to convert ferric ammonium citrate to an iron oxide. The iron oxide is visible as a reddish-brown or rust color on the colonies. In this illustration, the tube on the left is the negative control; the center tube, inoculated with *M. chelonae*, is negative; and the tube on the right, inoculated with *M. fortuitum*, is the positive control.

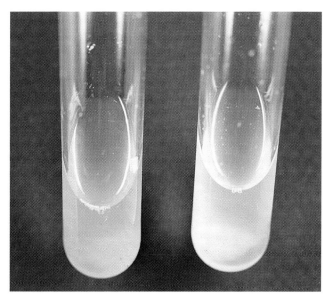

**11-26 Niacin accumulation test.** Most strains of *M. tuberculosis, M. simiae,* and some strains of Bacille Calmette-Guérin, the attenuated vaccine strain of *M. bovis*, excrete niacin into the culture medium. Reagent paper strips impregnated with substrates are used to test for niacin, which reacts with a cyanogen halide in the presence of a primary amine to produce a yellow color. In this example, in which the paper strips were removed after color development, the tube on the left is positive (yellow) and the tube on the right is negative (colorless).

# CHAPTER 12  Microbial Pathogens Isolated and/or Identified by Tissue Culture or Other Special Methods

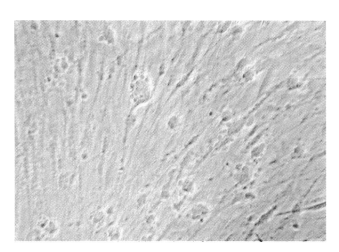 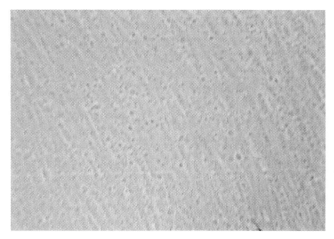

**12-1, 2 *Clostridium difficile*. Cytotoxin cell culture assay using MRC-5 cells. Phase contrast microscopy (×225).** Culture for *C. difficile* is a highly sensitive technique but not very specific, since this bacterium can be present in asymptomatic individuals. For this reason, the tissue culture assay for the detection of the *C. difficile* cytotoxin B is one recommended laboratory diagnostic method. Figure 12-1 shows the toxic effect produced by fecal supernatants containing toxin added to the MRC-5 monolayer, while Figure 12-2 shows a control monolayer, in which neutralizing antisera to the toxin B has been added, preventing development of the cytopathic effect.

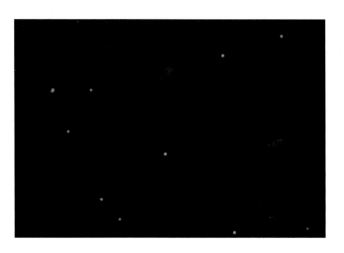

**12-3 *Chlamydia trachomatis*. Direct fluorescent assay (DFA) of cervical cells (×1250).** To perform this assay, cells from the endocervical os are collected with a swab, placed on a glass slide, and fixed with acetone. A fluorescein-labeled specific antibody is then added and the specimen is examined using a fluorescent microscope. In this figure, *C. trachomatis* elementary bodies have been stained with a monoclonal antibody to the outer membrane protein.

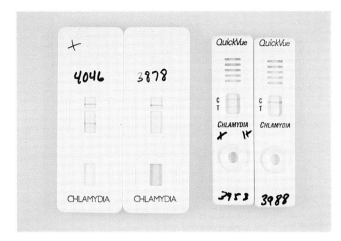

**12-4** *Chlamydia trachomatis.* **Direct antigen detection.** There are several commercially available filter-based enzyme immunoassay systems for the direct detection of *C. trachomatis.* For each of the two assays depicted here, the specimen is placed in the lower window of the card. The antigen migrates through the filter and binds to a chlamydial-specific antibody located on a line in the filter at the level of the second window. A positive reaction results in the formation of a color line (see cards on the left side for each system). Another antibody located in the filter at a greater distance from the specimen window is used as a control to ensure that the specimen has migrated through the filter.

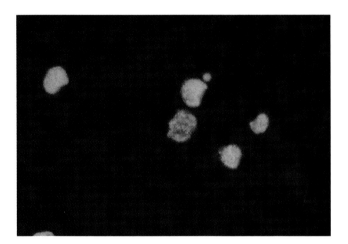

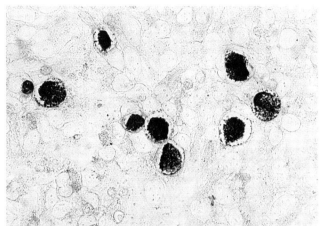

**12-5, 6** *Chlamydia trachomatis.* **Shell vial culture. Fluorescent and horseradish peroxidase stains (×500).** Shell vials with McCoy or HeLa cells are frequently used for the isolation of *C. trachomatis* from clinical specimens. Following centrifugation of the sample onto the cells, the cell monolayers are incubated for 48 hours. If viable *Chlamydia* were present in the sample, they will multiply in the cells of the monolayer and produce intracellular inclusions. The fixed inclusions can be stained with a fluorescein-labeled monoclonal antibody (Figure 12-5) or with an antibody labeled with horseradish peroxidase (Figure 12-6). A similar approach can be used for the detection of *Chlamydia pneumoniae* and *Chlamydia psittaci.*

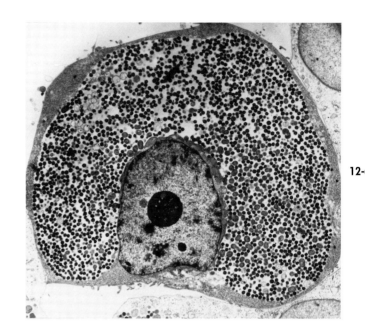

12-

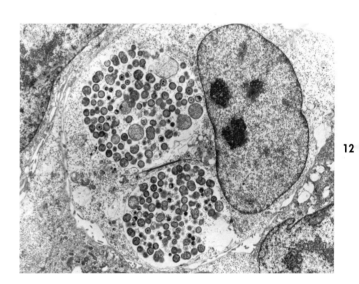

12

**12-7-9** *Chlamydia trachomatis* **and** *Chlamydia pneumoniae.* **Infected tissue culture cells viewed by transmission electron microscopy.** Large intracytoplasmic inclusions are formed by *Chlamydia* after 24 to 72 hours of intracellular growth. The elementary bodies are the mature infectious form of the organism and are dense, compact, and measure approximately 300 nm in diameter. The reticulate bodies are the replicative form, have a loose structure, and measure up to 1000 nm in diameter. Characteristically the inclusions of *C. trachomatis* surround the nucleus of the host cell (*Chlamydia:* from the Greek "chlamydion" meaning short mantel) (Figure 12-7; ×2750). *C. pneumoniae* may form multiple inclusions (Figure 12-8; ×2750). Some of the elementary bodies of *C. pneumoniae* may have a pyriform shape (Figure 12-9; ×35,500).

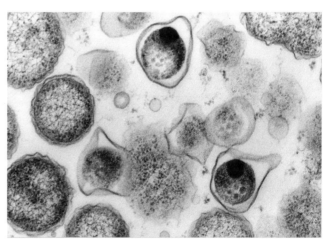

12

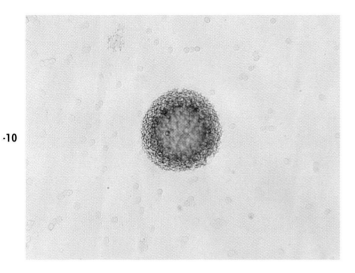

-10

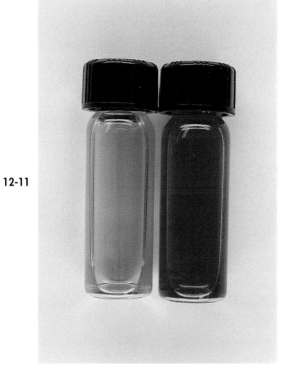

12-11

**12-10-12** *Mycoplasma and Ureaplasma species.* Mycoplasmas are the smallest free-living organisms. Unlike classic bacteria they lack a cell wall and behave as parasites on the surface of the host cells but are not intracellular. Complex media and tissue culture techniques are used for their isolation. *Ureaplasma urealyticum* were originally named T (tiny) mycoplasmas due to the small size of their colonies, usually 15 to 30 μm in diameter (Figure 12-10; viewed through a light microscope). *U. urealyticum* induces an alkaline color change (purple) without turbidity in a medium that contains urea (Figure 12-11, *left tube;* control tube is on the right). The genital mycoplasmas grow better in 5% $CO_2$ and produce the typical fried-egg appearance morphology (Figure 12-12 shows *M. hominis* colonies viewed through a light microscope).

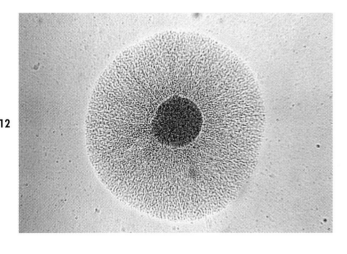

12

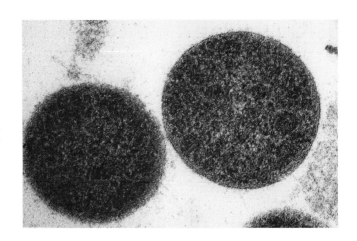

**12-13** *Ureaplasma urealyticum.* **Transmission electron microscopy (×77,000).** The ultrastructure of the mycoplasmas and ureaplasmas is pleomorphic and fairly indistinct. They measure 200 to 300 nm in diameter and have a cell membrane, but they do not have a cell wall.

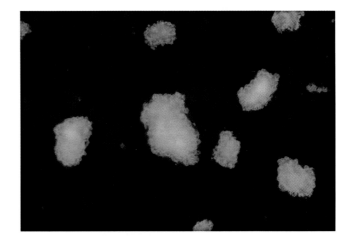

**12-14 Mycoplasmas and ureaplasmas. Antibody detection by microimmunofluorescence (MIF) test.** There are several approaches, including complement fixation, metabolic inhibition, and fluorescence assays, for detecting antibodies to these microorganisms. For the MIF test, the serum of the patient is reacted with colonies of mycoplasma present on the slide, and antihuman fluorescein-labeled globulin is then added. This test is fairly specific and sensitive and allows for the detection of IgM as well as IgG antibodies.

# CHAPTER 13 *Antimicrobial Susceptibility Testing (AST)*

Numerous antimicrobial susceptibility test procedures have been described. Qualitative tests, such as the agar disk diffusion method, categorize the bacterial isolate as susceptible, intermediate, and resistant. Quantitative methods are used to determine a specific endpoint, referred to as the minimal inhibitory concentration (MIC; the minimal amount of antimicrobial agent that inhibits visible growth).

In the disk diffusion method, used for rapidly growing aerobic bacteria, a standardized pure culture inoculum is swabbed onto the surface of a Mueller-Hinton agar plate. Filter paper disks impregnated with antimicrobial agents are placed on the agar plate. After overnight incubation, the zone of inhibited growth surrounding each disk is measured and results are compared to guidelines published by the National Committee for Clinical Laboratory Standards (NCCLS; Wayne, Pa.).

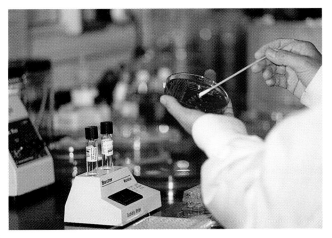

**13-1 Preparation of standardized inoculum.** Three to five colonies of similar morphology are selected on a cotton swab from a fresh, 18- to 24-hour culture and transferred into 4 to 5 ml Mueller-Hinton broth or trypticase soy broth. Either the broth is incubated for 2 to 8 hours or the selected colonies are inoculated into 0.85% sterile saline or broth without incubation to produce a suspension of the desired turbidity. The direct method is preferred for those microorganisms that are fastidious and have unpredictable growth in broth.

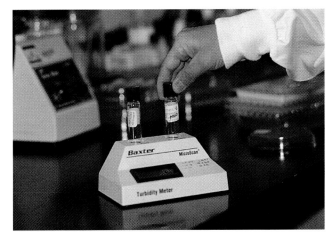

**13-2 Using a turbidity meter to adjust the inoculum.** The suspension is vortex mixed for 15 to 20 seconds before determining its turbidity. A meter is used to adjust the inoculum to a 0.5 McFarland turbidity standard, which is equal to approximately $1.5 \times 10^8$ colony forming units (CFU) per ml. The turbidity is adjusted to match the standard by diluting with additional saline or broth.

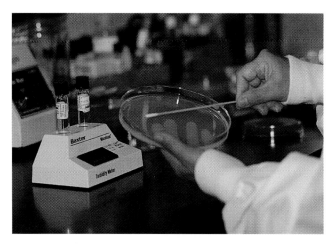

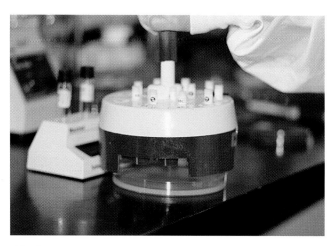

**13-3  Disk diffusion method—Agar plate inoculation.** A sterile cotton swab is dipped into the inoculum and the entire surface of the Mueller-Hinton agar plate is swabbed three times by rotating the plate approximately 60° between streaking to ensure even distribution. The plate is allowed to stand for at least 3 minutes, but no longer than 15 minutes, before applying the disks.

**13-4  Disk diffusion method—application of disks.** Disks are applied to the agar surface using a dispenser. No more than 12 disks should be placed on a 150 mm plate. A disk should not be relocated once it has made contact with the agar surface because antimicrobial diffusion begins immediately. Agar plates must be incubated within 15 minutes of disk application.

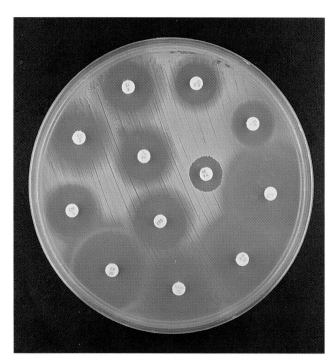

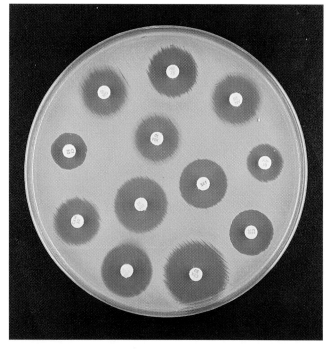

**13-5  Disk diffusion method—*Staphylococcus aureus* American Type Culture Collection (ATCC) 25923.** The zone of growth inhibition is measured using a millimeter ruler or calipers. Results are interpreted as susceptible (S), intermediate (I), or resistant (R). The size of the disk (6 mm) is included in the measurement; therefore, those agents with no zone are measured as 6 mm and are always interpreted as resistant. The microorganism tested on this Mueller-Hinton agar plate is susceptible to all antimicrobial agents.

**13-6  Disk diffusion method—*Escherichia coli* ATCC 25922.** The isolate tested on this Mueller-Hinton agar plate is interpreted as susceptible (S) to all antimicrobial agents. Reading clockwise from the top, they are mezlocillin (MZ), amikacin (AN), ampicillin (AM), cefazolin (CZ), cefotaxime (CTX), cefuroxime (CXM), cephalothin (CF), gentamicin (GM), and tobramycin (NN); the three disks in the center of the plate are trimethoprim/sulfamethoxazole (SXT), cefoxitin (FOX), and ticarcillin/clavulanic acid (TIM).

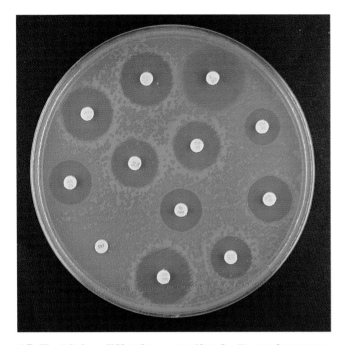

**13-7 Disk diffusion method—*Pseudomonas aeruginosa* ATCC 27853.** On this Mueller-Hinton agar plate, the isolate is resistant to trimethoprim/sulfamethoxazole (SXT) and susceptible to all others; they include ciprofloxacin (CIP), gentamicin (GM), amikacin (AN), aztreonam (ATM), ticarcillin/clavulanic acid (TIM), tobramycin (NN), ticarcillin (TIC), mezlocillin (MZ), ceftazidime (CAZ), imipenem (IPM), and piperacillin (PIP).

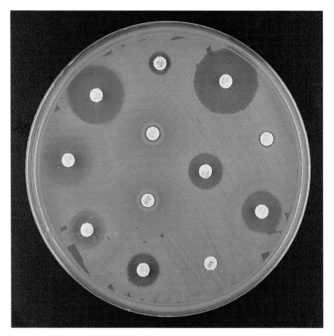

**13-8 Disk diffusion method—*Pseudomonas aeruginosa*, a resistant strain.** Growth on this Mueller-Hinton agar plate indicates that the isolate is resistant to six of the 12 antimicrobial agents and susceptible to the remaining. The isolate is resistant to trimethoprim/sulfamethoxazole (SXT), gentamicin (GM), aztreonam (ATM), ticarcillin/clavulanic acid (TIM), ticarcillin (TIC), and mezlocillin (MZ). The isolate is susceptible to ciprofloxacin (CIP), amikacin (AN), tobramycin (NN), ceftazidime (CAZ), imipenem (IPM), and piperacillin (PIP).

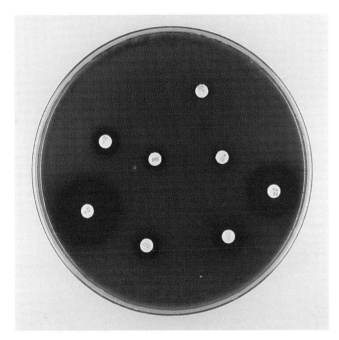

**13-9 Disk diffusion method—*Streptococcus pneumoniae*—secondary test battery when oxacillin is resistant (less than 20 mm) to oxacillin.** *S. pneumoniae* on Mueller-Hinton agar with 5% sheep blood. The isolate is susceptible to vancomycin (VA) and rifampin (RA) and intermediate to clindamycin (CC). The isolate is resistant to the remaining agents oxacillin (OX), erythromycin (E), tetracycline (TE), chloramphenicol (C), and trimethoprim/sulfamethoxazole (SXT).

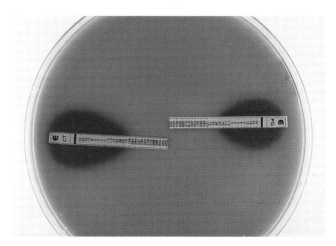

**13-10 E test method—*Streptococcus pneumoniae*.** The E test (AB Biodisk North America, Inc., Piscataway, NJ) uses strips impregnated with an antibiotic gradient to determine the MIC of an organism. After overnight incubation, a symmetrical inhibition ellipse is formed. The zone edge intersects the strip at the MIC value given in µg/ml. In this example, the MIC of penicillin G (PG) is 0.5 µg/ml (intermediate); the MIC of ceftriaxone (CT) is 0.125 µg/ml (susceptible).

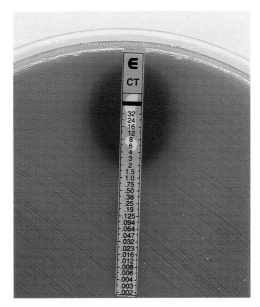

**13-11  E test method—*Streptococcus pneumoniae.*** In this figure, the MIC of cefotaxime (CT) is between 1.5 µg/ml and 2.0 µg/ml. The MIC should be reported as 2.0 µg/ml, which is interpreted as resistant.

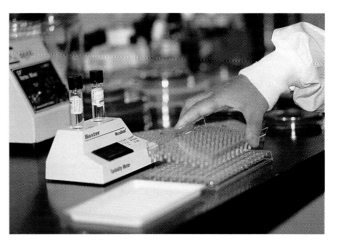

**13-12  Broth Microdilution Method—Inoculation of microdilution panel.** Microdilution panels are used to quantitatively measure the susceptibility of microorganisms to a battery of antimicrobial agents. The inoculum is mixed and poured into the inoculum/seed tray. The inoculator tips are lowered into the tray and the tips filled by capillary action. The inoculator tips are then lowered into the wells of the panel, as shown here.

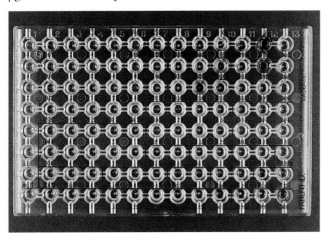

**13-13  Broth Microdilution Method—Inoculated microdilution panel.** This Pasco microdilution panel (Difco Laboratories, Detroit, Mich.) includes wells for both identification biochemicals and quantitative antimicrobial susceptibility testing. If all antimicrobial dilutions show inhibition of growth, the endpoint is less than or equal to the lowest concentration tested, assuming that the positive growth control exhibits growth. Interpretation is based on NCCLS approved standards.

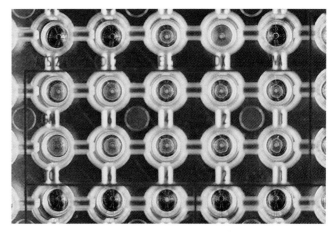

**13-14  Broth Microdilution Method—interpretation of microdilution panel.** Close-up view of 20 wells of the microdilution panel. Note the drug name and concentration in blue ink directly below the corresponding well. Row 1, left to right, the antimicrobics and interpretations are as follows:  ampicillin/sulbactam (A/S) - no growth (MIC≤2/1 µg/ml); clindamycin (CD) - no growth (MIC≤2 µg/ml); erythromycin (E) - growth (MIC >0.5 µg/ml); oxacillin (OX) - growth (MIC >1 µg/ml); vancomycin (VA) - no growth (MIC ≤2 µg/ml).

Row 2, gentamicin (GM) - interpretation: growth in all 5 wells, MIC is >8 µg/ml.

Row 3, tobramycin (TO) - interpretation: growth in all 5 wells, MIC is >8 µg/ml.

Row 4, wells 1 to 3, ceftriaxone (FRX) - dilutions, left to right, 32, 16, and 8 µg/ml. Interpretation: growth in 8 µg/ml, no growth in 16 and 32 µg/ml; MIC is 16 µg/ml.

Row 4, wells 4 and 5, chloramphenicol (C) - dilutions, left to right, 16 and 8 µg/ml. Interpretation: no growth in either well, MIC is 8 µg/ml.

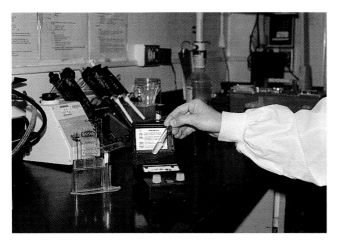

**13-15 Automated method—Preparation of standardized inoculum.** Several instruments for automated performance of ASTs are available. Preparation of inoculum for the Vitek (bioMerieux Vitek, Inc., Hazelwood, Mo) system is performed using the bioMerieux Vitek colorimeter, a single-beam photometer with a 450 nm filter. The inoculum suspension is vortexed and the turbidity is measured as shown in this slide.

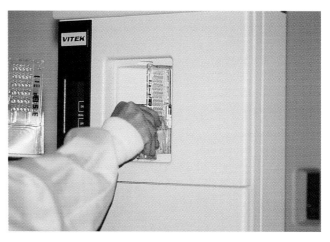

**13-16 Automated method—sealing the Vitek card.** The standardized inoculum and the card containing the diluted antimicrobics are first placed into the filling module of the Vitek instrument. Once the inoculum is transferred into the card by vacuum suction through the plastic transfer tube, the card is sealed in the sealing module, as shown here.

A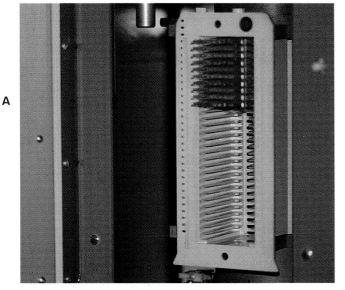

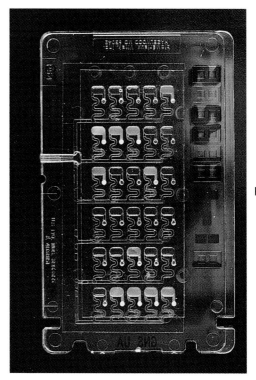 B

**13-17 A, Automated method—Vitek card in the reader incubator.** Once the card has been sealed, the card is inspected for a proper fill and then it is placed into the reader incubator as shown here. The results are determined by the electro-optical detection of microbial growth within wells of the test cards. MICs are determined by statistical analysis of bacterial growth rates in the presence of antimicrobial agents. **B, Incubated Vitek card.** This Vitek Gram-negative susceptibility card (GNS-UA) is used for performing ASTs on gram-negative isolates from urine specimens. Once the growth control well reaches the turbidity threshold, the instrument reads the remaining wells, which contain various dilutions of antimicrobics. In this slide, turbid wells (resistant) are shown in five of the six rows, while only clear wells (susceptible) are shown in the fourth row.

**13-18 Detection of beta-lactamase production by cefinase.** Beta-lactamase enzymes produced by bacteria break down penicillins and render the producing strains resistant to penicillins. The method shown here detects all known beta-lactamases. The cefinase disk (Becton Dickinson Microbiology Systems, Cockeysville, Md.) is impregnated with nitrocefin, a chromogenic cephalosporin. Colonies of the microorganism are rubbed onto the disk. If the amide bond in the nitrocefin beta-lactam ring is hydrolyzed by a beta-lactamase enzyme from the microorganism, the color of the disk will rapidly change from yellow to red.

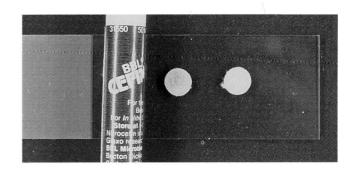

**13-19 Positive beta-lactamase test.** The pink color on the surface of the disk that was inoculated with the test microorganism indicates the presence of beta-lactamase. This test is used to determine beta-lactamase activity in staphylococci, *Haemophilus influenzae*, *Moraxella catarrhalis*, *Neisseria gonorrhoeae*, *Neisseria meningitidis*, enterococci, and certain anaerobic bacteria including *Bacteroides* spp.

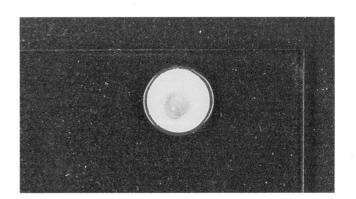

**13-20 Schlichter test/serum inhibitory titer.** Determining the activity of an antimicrobial agent in the patient's serum may be useful in certain infections requiring prolonged antimicrobial therapy, such as endocarditis and osteomyelitis. For the Schlichter test, the patient's serum containing an antimicrobial agent is inoculated with the patient's own infecting microorganism. After incubation, the inhibitory titer is interpreted as the highest dilution of the serum showing no visible growth, as shown on the far left tube, while the other three tubes illustrate growth of the microorganism.

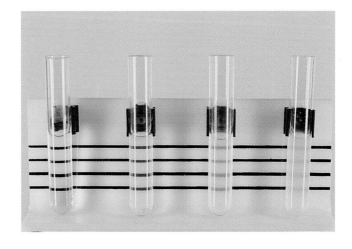

# CHAPTER 14 *Mycology*

I dentification of fungi is still based largely on gross and microscopic morphological characteristics. In addition to visual inspection, commercially available biochemical manual or automated systems, nucleic acid probes, and serological reagents are used. The fungi are broadly divided into yeast, characterized by opaque, creamy colonies, and molds that produce cottony or powdery growth. Some species, particularly some that cause systemic infection, are dimorphic and can assume either morphotype.

This section presents the agents of fungal infections in a commonly used clinical classification. Systemic or deep-seated mycoses often begin in the respiratory tract and disseminate. Subcutaneous mycoses are frequently secondary to traumatic implantation. Systemic spread of these infections is less likely. Superficial infections are confined to the keratinous layer of skin, nails, and hair and in general there is minimal host inflammatory response. The "opportunistic mycoses" usually cause infections only in immunocompromised hosts. The causative fungi are common environmental inhabitants. The "miscellaneous" category includes those fungal infections that do not fit easily into the other headings.

## Deep-seated Mycoses

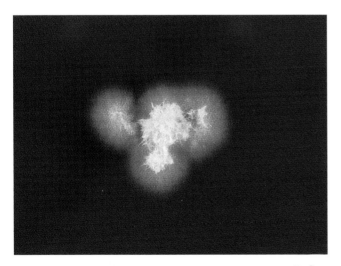

**14-1 *Blastomyces dermatitidis* colonies.** B. dermatitidis growing on brain heart infusion agar with 10% sheep blood, gentamicin, and chloramphenicol. At 25°C the mold form of *B. dermatitidis* produces white to tan, cottony colonies that grow fairly rapidly in a week. With age they turn dark brown. At 37°C the yeast form produces cream to brown, wrinkled, waxy-looking colonies (not shown).

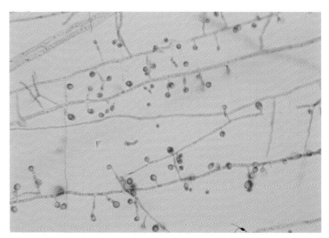

**14-2 *Blastomyces dermatitidis* mycelial phase. Lactophenol cotton blue preparation (×500).** As shown here, at 25°C in the mold form, the conidia of *B. dermatitidis* are round to oval, with a hyaline smooth wall, and are attached to short lateral or terminal hyphal branches giving the appearance of "lollipops." The conidia measure 2 to 10 μm in diameter.

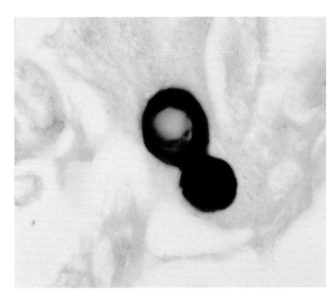

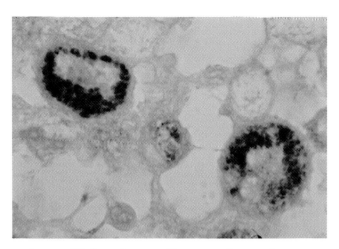

**14-3, 4 Yeast form of *Blastomyces dermatitidis*. Lung tissue. Gomori methenamine silver stain (Figure 14-3, ×1850; Figure 14-4, ×1250).** At 37°C the yeast form of *B. dermatitidis* appears as thick-walled, spherical cells with a wide-based single bud (Figure 14-3). Small forms may occasionally emerge, particularly in tissue, which cannot be easily differentiated from *H. capsulatum* (Figure 14-4).

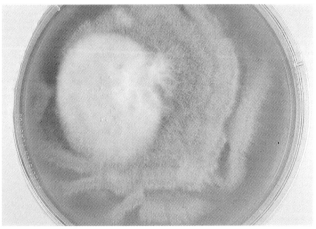

**14-5 *Coccidioides immitis* growing on Sabouraud's dextrose agar.** *C. immitis* grows well on Sabouraud's medium at 25°C. Within 1 or 2 weeks, the gray-tan colony has a powdery, cottony appearance resulting from the formation of arthroconidia from the hyphae. The colony becomes tan to brown with age, and the reverse side is white. Other colony colors are seen occasionally.

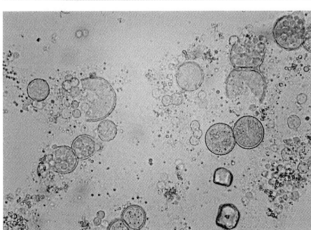

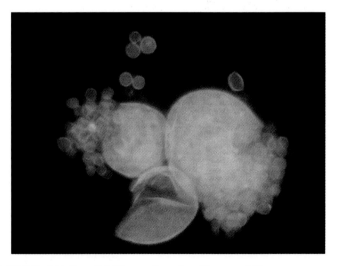

**14-6, 7 *Coccidioides immitis* wet mount (KOH; 14-6, ×500), and calcofluor white (14-7, ×1200) preparations.** Mature spherules of *C. immitis* are round or oval, measure 15 to 60 μm in diameter, have a well demarcated wall, and produce endospores by undergoing progressive cleavage. The endospores measure 2 to 5 μm in diameter, do not bud, and are extruded from the mature spherules. Once they are extruded, the endospores initiate maturation, becoming spherules that eventually undergo cleavages that result in new endospores. It is important to recognize that immature spherules that lack endospores can be mistaken for other fungi, such as *Blastomyces dermatitidis*, and for artifacts.

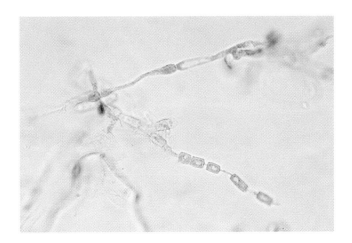

**14-8 Lactophenol cotton blue preparation of arthroconidia of *Coccidioides immitis* (×500).** The arthroconidia of *C. immitis* appear in the branches of the hyphae as thick-walled, barrel-shaped structures measuring 4 to 6 by 2 to 4 μm. Alternating with the arthroconidia are weakly stained empty cells, a characteristic that differentiates this microorganism from *Geotrichum* spp. The arthroconidia mature, break off, and following aspiration they can produce an infection in susceptible individuals.

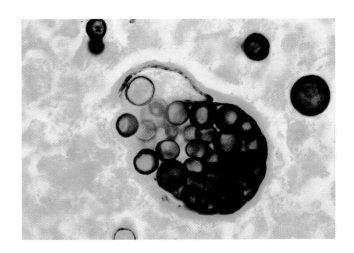

**14-9 Tissue section of the lung stained with Gomori's methenamine silver showing a *Coccidioides immitis* spherule (×1250).** The wall of the spherule has ruptured and the endospores are released into the surrounding tissues. In general, the walls of the endospores stain darker than the walls of the spherules. Spherules that lack endospores need to be differentiated from other fungi including *Histoplasma capsulatum*, *Torulopsis (Candida) glabrata*, *Cryptococcus neoformans*, and *Paracoccidioides brasiliensis*.

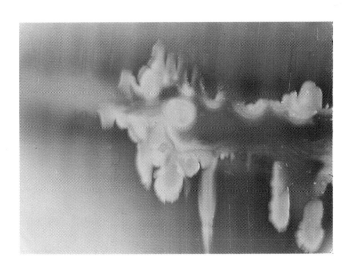

**14-10 *Cryptococcus neoformans* colonies growing on chocolate agar.** The colonies of *C. neoformans* are typically flat or slightly raised, shiny, mucoid as a result of the presence of a mucopolysaccharide capsule, and may have a wide variation in color ranging from cream to tan and pink. With age, the colonies tend to become drier and darker in color.

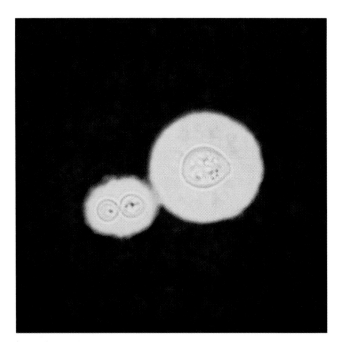

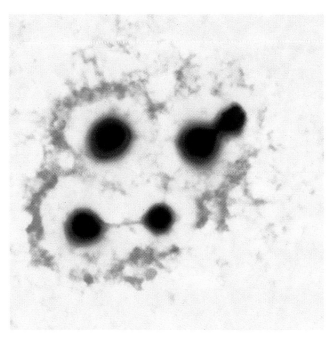

**14-11, 12   India ink (14-11) and Gram stain (14-12) preparations of *Cryptococcus neoformans* (×2250).** The cells shown here are surrounded by a broad mucopolysaccharide capsule. The thickness of the capsule can vary widely from preparation to preparation, and in certain instances the capsule may be undetectable using India ink. The cells are round to oval, with a diameter ranging from 3 to 10 μm, and have a single bud with a narrow neck. The India ink preparation is not as sensitive as the latex agglutination antigen detection tests for initial detection of *C. neoformans* in cerebrospinal fluid. Specimens negative by India ink should be tested for antigen; all cerebrospinal fluid specimens sent for India ink preparation should also be cultured.

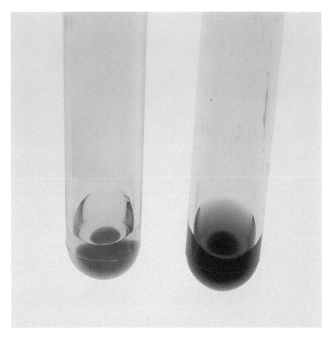

**14-13   Urease test for *Cryptococcus neoformans*.** Over 99% of the *C. neoformans* isolates give a positive urease test, pink-purple color, within 15 minutes, in contrast to other urease-positive species of yeast that require more than 3 hours to give a positive reaction.

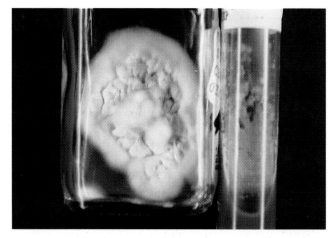

**14-14   Colonies of *Histoplasma capsulatum*.** Note the yeast form of *H. capsulatum* growing on chocolate agar at 37°C (*right side*), and the mycelial form growing on Sabouraud's dextrose agar at 25°C (*left side*). The yeast form appears waxy and moist with a yellow-tan color, while the mycelial form has a cottony appearance with a white-brown or pinkish color.

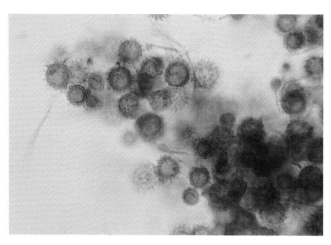

**14-15 Lactophenol cotton blue stained *Histoplasma capsulatum* (×500).** After several days in culture at 25°C, thick-walled, tuberculate (knobby), and nontuberculate macroconidia appear, measuring 10 to 15 μm in diameter. The microconidia of *H. capsulatum* emerge during the early stages of colony growth as spherical or oval structures, 3 to 5 μm in diameter.

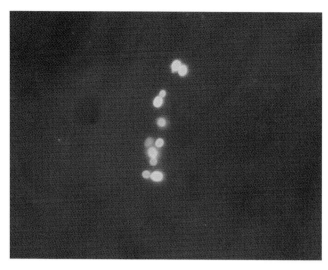

**14-16 Direct bone marrow preparation showing *Histoplasma capsulatum* stained with calcofluor white (×2500).** Round to oval, small, 2 × 5 μm, narrow-based, budding yeast cells can be observed on this direct bone marrow preparation.

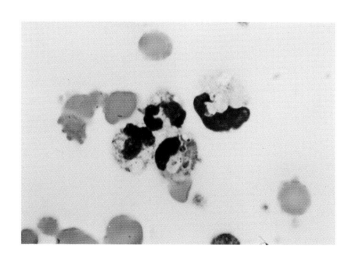

**14-17 Buffy coat preparation showing *Histoplasma capsulatum* (×1250).** White blood cells containing blastoconidia of *H. capsulatum*. The budding yeast seems to be surrounded by a capsule. This pseudocapsule is thought to be an artifact resulting from shrinking tissues during fixation.

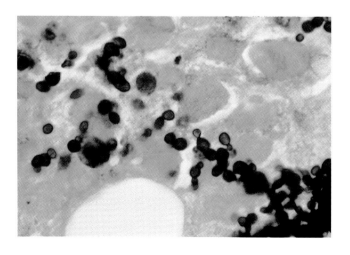

**14-18 Lung section showing *Histoplasma capsulatum* stained with Gomori's methenamine silver (×1250).** The yeast form of *H. capsulatum* is usually found intracellularly in the cytoplasm of professional phagocytes. The microorganism is elongated, measures approximately 2 to 5 μm, and multiplies by narrow-based, unequal budding.

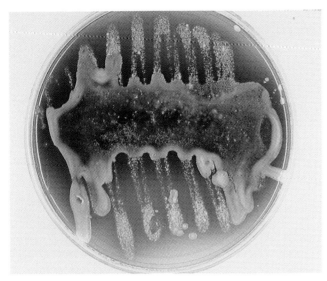

**14-19   Mixed culture of *Histoplasma capsulatum* and *Cryptococcus neoformans.*** This patient had a double infection, and thus colonies of both *H. capsulatum* and *C. neoformans* are growing on this plate. This possibility should be taken into consideration, particularly in specimens from patients that are immunocompromised. Plates should be incubated for at least 4 weeks and should not be discarded earlier, even when a rapid grower is already present.

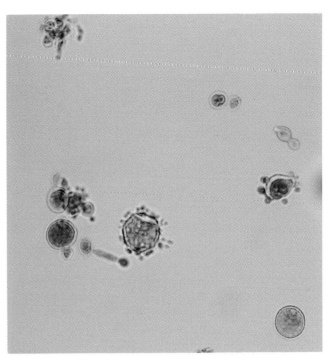

**14-20   *Paracoccidioides brasiliensis* stained with lactophenol cotton blue (×325).** In this preparation, cultured at 37°C, large, thick-walled cells with multiple buddings are attached to the mother cells by narrow connections, giving the characteristic appearance of a "ship's wheel" or "steering wheel." At 25°C most strains grow for a long time without producing conidia. There are different types of conidia that may form, none of which is characteristic of this species.

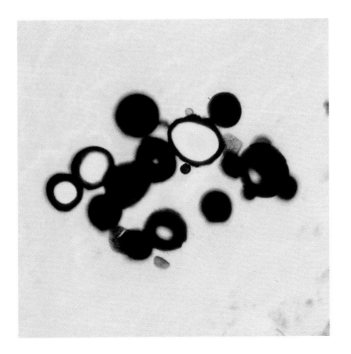

**14-21   *Paracoccidioides brasiliensis.* Adrenal tissue. Gomori's methenamine silver stain (×500).** This preparation demonstrates numerous thick-walled yeast cells, spherical to oval, measuring up to 60 to 70 μm in diameter with multiple narrow-based buds that give the typical appearance of a "steering wheel" and "Mickey Mouse" type forms.

# Opportunistic Mycoses

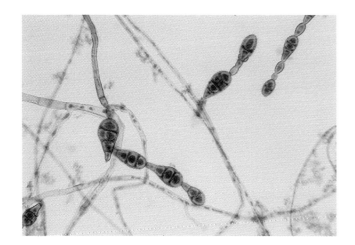

**14-22 Lactophenol cotton blue preparation of *Alternaria* spp. (×500).** The mycelia are septate and dark. The conidiophores produce tan-brown conidia that are large, approximately $10 \times 30$ μm, round at the end near the conidiophore, and narrow at the far end giving a clavate (clublike) shape, with a smooth or rough wall, and transverse and longitudinal septations.

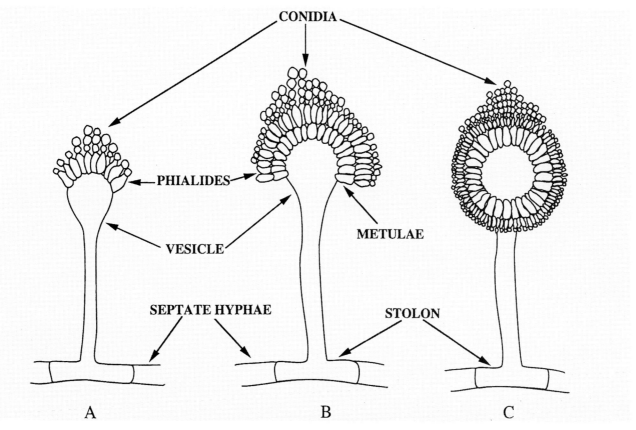

**14-23 Diagram of the morphological structure of *Aspergillus* spp.** *Aspergillus fumigatus* **(A)** is uniseriate (e.g., has only one layer of phialides that cover the upper two-thirds of the vesicle). The phialides bear the conidia, which are extruded from the end of the unconstricted phialide. *Aspergillus versicolor* **(B)** and *A. niger* **(C)** are biseriate, in which the vesicle is covered with a layer of short hyphal structures called metulae (the structures bearing the phialides) and another layer consisting of the phialides. The metulae and phialides of *A. niger* form a radiate arrangement **(C)** but those of *A. versicolor* do not **(B)**. *Aspergillus flavus* may be both uniseriate and biseriate with the metulae and phialides covering the entire vesicle.

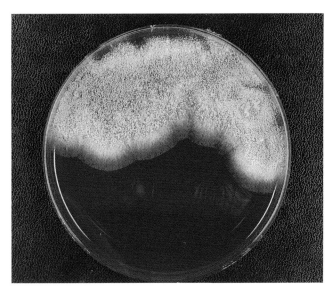

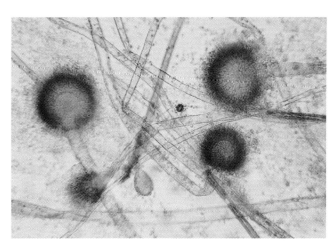

**14-24 Colonies of *Aspergillus flavus* growing on a sheep blood agar plate.** The colonies of *A. flavus* have a distinct velvety yellow to yellow-green or brown color. The green-brown color is more prominent in older cultures. The reverse is white to red-brown. This microorganism grows better at 37°C than at room temperature.

**14-25 Lactophenol cotton blue preparation of *Aspergillus flavus* (×225).** The conidial heads measure approximately 300 to 400 μm in diameter and may have uniseriate and biseriate rows of phialides that cover the entire vesicle. Usually the proximal row of sterigmata is twice the length of the outer row. The conidia do not usually chain and tend to accumulate over the vesicle.

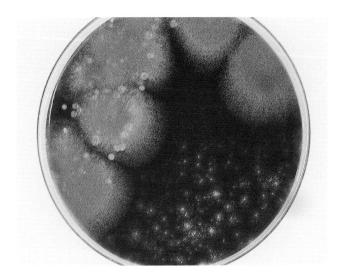

**14-26 *Aspergillus fumigatus* growing on a sheep blood agar plate.** The colonies of *A. fumigatus* grow well at 20 to 43°C. Incubating the specimens of *A. fumigatus* at temperatures above 43°C helps to inhibit the growth of contaminants. The color of the colonies ranges from white to green and with age they tend to turn gray, brown, or black.

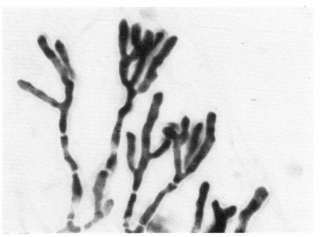

**14-27 Gram stain of *Aspergillus fumigatus* (×1250).** *A. fumigatus* typically appears as uniform septate hyphae with dichotomous (two-way) acute (45°C) branching. The hyphae have parallel walls without constrictions, and are fairly uniform in width, measuring 3 to 6 μm in diameter.

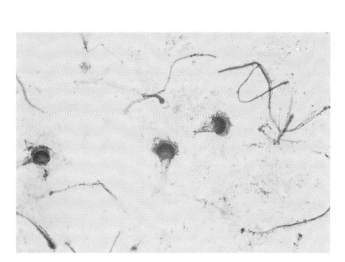

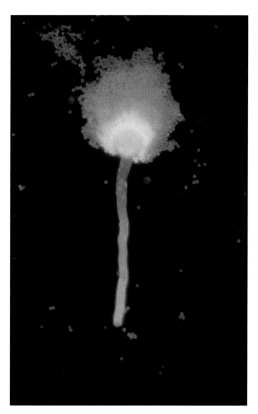

**14-28, 29** *Aspergillus fumigatus* **stained with lactophenol cotton blue (14-28 [×225]) or with calcofluor white (14-29 [×500]).** The conidiophore of *A. fumigatus* measures up to 300 to 500 μm in length and 4 to 8 μm in width. The vesicle is dome-shaped, 20 to 30 μm in diameter, and merges with the conidiophore. Phialides are present only in the upper half or two thirds of the vesicle and extend in the same direction as the conidiophore. The small, oval-round, green-tan conidia are borne in chains from the tips of the phialides or sterigmata.

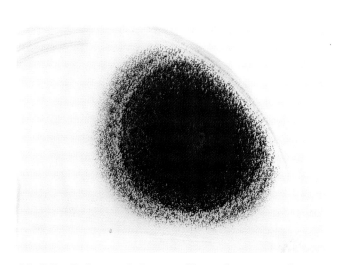

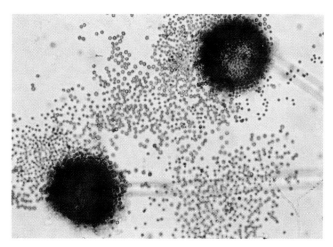

**14-30 Colony of** *Aspergillus niger* **growing on Sabouraud's dextrose agar.** *A. niger* colonies are fairly distinct, with a woolly appearance, originally displaying a white-yellow color that turns to dark brown-black due to the conidial heads, with a white to tan basal layer.

**14-31** *Aspergillus niger* **stained with lactophenol cotton blue (×500).** The conidiophores of *A. niger* are large, measuring up to 2 to 3 mm in length by 15 to 20 μm in width. The vesicle is globular, 40 to 80 μm in diameter, brown-black, with biseriate phialides that cover the entire surface of the vesicle forming a radiate head.

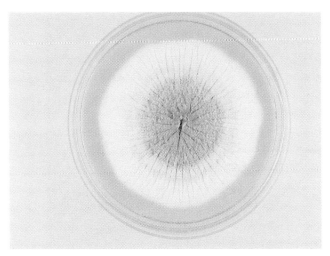

**14-32** *Aspergillus terreus* **colony on Sabouraud's dextrose agar.** This colony of *A. terreus* has a velvety white, cinnamon-buff to brown color on the surface, and is white to brown on the reverse side.

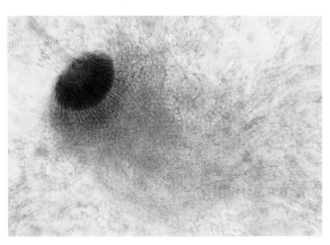

**14-33** *Aspergillus terreus* **stained with lactophenol cotton blue (×500).** The conidial heads of *A. terreus* measure up to 500 μm in diameter and are biseriate. The conidia are spherical to oval with a hyaline smooth wall and, as shown in this figure, can form long chains.

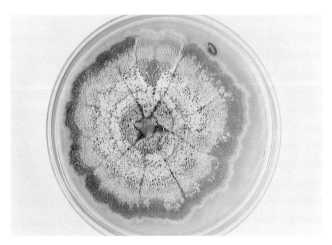

**14-34** *Aspergillus versicolor* **colony on Sabouraud's dextrose agar.** The colonies of *A. versicolor* usually display a wide range of colors including white-tan to yellow, green, and brown.

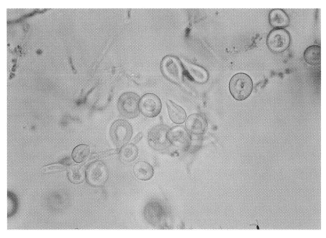

**14-35** *Aspergillus versicolor* **stained with lactophenol cotton blue (×1250).** This figure shows Hülle cells produced by *A. versicolor*. These structures are also produced by other species of aspergilli, and it is not clear what their function is. They are thick-walled, spherical or pear-shaped, and are produced as terminal or intercalary cells on the hyphae.

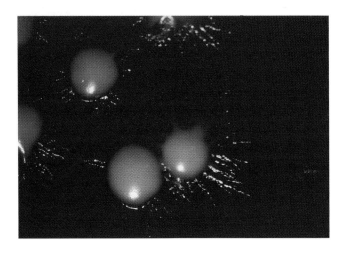

**14-36** *Candida albicans* **growing on sheep blood agar plates.** The colonies of *C. albicans* are white or tan, opaque, smooth, and as shown in this figure, may have small extensions or "feet" that increase with the age of the colony. The colonies grow rapidly and can usually be detected in 24 to 48 hours when grown aerobically at 25 to 30°C.

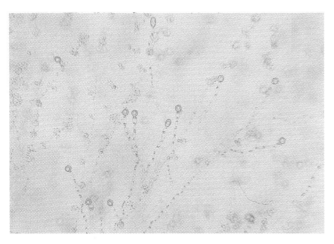

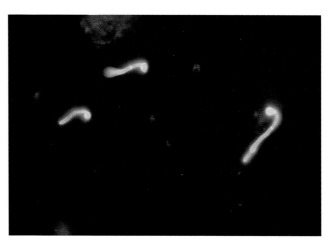

**14-37** *Candida albicans* **grown on a corn meal agar with trypan blue.** As shown in this figure, *C. albicans* grown at 25°C for 48 to 72 hours forms septate pseudohyphae with groups of blastospores at the septa, and large thick-walled terminal chlamydospores that are typical of this species.

**14-38** *Candida albicans* **germ tubes stained with calcofluor white (×625).** A simple test for the identification of *C. albicans* is the germ tube test. Part of a colony is emulsified in fetal bovine serum and incubated at 37°C for 2 to 3 hours. The germ tubes are approximately half the width and two to four times the length of the yeast cells. The germ tubes produced by *C. albicans* are not constricted at the union with the blastoconidium as is the case with *Candida tropicalis.*

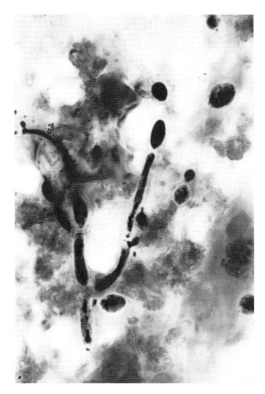

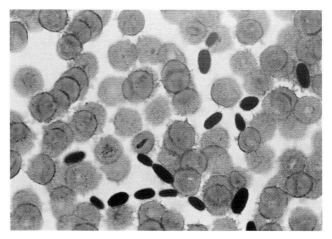

**14-39** *Candida albicans.* **Blood culture. Gram stain (×1350).** Blood culture from a patient with a *C. albicans* fungemia. Blastoconidia can be observed budding and producing the pseudohyphae. The blastoconidia stain gram-positive, are round or oval, and measure approximately 3 × 5 μm.

**14-40** *Candida tropicalis.* **Blood culture. Gram stain (×1250).** The blastoconidia of *C. tropicalis* tend to be more barrel-shaped and irregular than those of *C. albicans.*

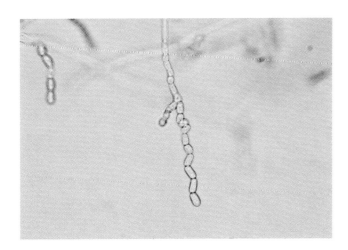

**14-41** *Geotrichum* **sp. grown on corn meal agar with trypan blue.** Chains of smooth, hyaline, cylindrical arthroconidia with round corners, are characteristic of this species. The arthrocondia originate by segmentation of the hyphae, and typically they germinate from one corner, giving the appearance of a "hockey stick." The formation of consecutive arthroconidia differentiates this genus from *Coccidioides immitis*.

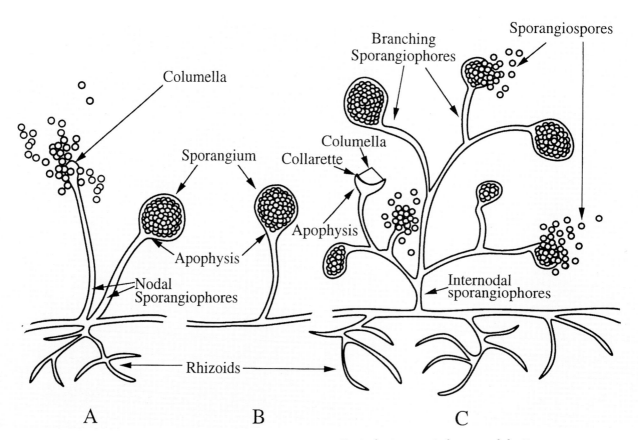

**14-42 Diagram of *Zygomycetes* structure.** Typical microscopic features of the *Zygomycetes*, a group with generally aseptate hyphae, are shown here. The organisms of the *Rhizopus* spp. **(A)** have nodal sporangiophores, e.g., rhizoids (root-like structures) are formed at the point where the sporangiophores meet the stolon (horizontal section of hyphae from which sporangiophores and rhizoids arise). No rhizoids are found in the *Mucor* spp. **(B)**. *Absidia* spp. **(C)** form internodal sporangiophores. When the wall of the sporangium breaks, a collarette remains at the top of the sporangiophore and the pointed columella becomes visible.

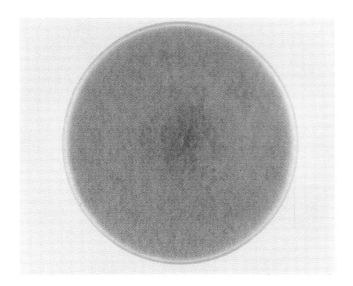

**14-43** *Absidia corymbifera* **colony in Sabouraud's dextrose agar.** The colonies of *A. corymbifera* grow rapidly, filling the Petri dish, and have a woolly, white color that turns gray with age. The reverse side is white. In general, all colonies of *Zygomycetes* have similar colony characteristics.

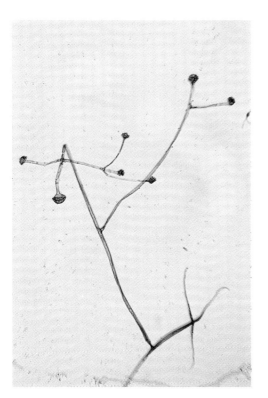

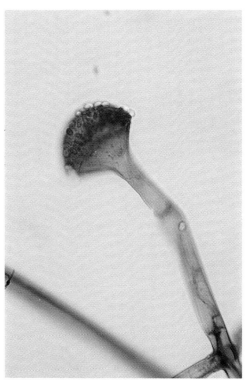

**14-44, 45 Lactophenol cotton blue preparations of** *Absidia corymbifera* **(14-44, ×80; 14-45, ×550).** *A. corymbifera* produces few rhizoids and, in contrast to those of the genus *Rhizopus*, the sporangiophores grow at a point on the stolon that is between the rhizoids and not opposite them. The sporangiophores are characteristically highly branched (Figure 14-44). The sporangium of *A. corymbifera* has a pyriform shape, small size, measuring 20 to 40 μm in diameter, with a conical columella and a distinct apophysis (Figure 14-45). The sporangiospores are oval in shape, measure approximately 3 × 5 μm and have a smooth wall.

**14-46 *Mucor* spp. stained with lactophenol cotton blue (×500).** The sporangiophores of *Mucor* spp. have terminal spherical sporangia that measure up to 300 μm in diameter, containing numerous round sporangiospores. The sporangiophores are hyaline, smooth, with a gray-tan color, and they do not have apophyses. The columella is well developed and has a prominent collarette at the junction with the sporangiophore. No rhizoids are found in this species.

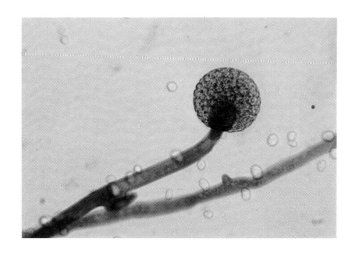

**14-47 *Mucor* spp. Lung. Gomori's methenamine silver stain (×1250).** In tissues, the hyphae of *Mucor* spp. are broad, irregular, with bulbous lateral protrusions, and do not have septae; branching occurs preferentially at wide angles (90°).

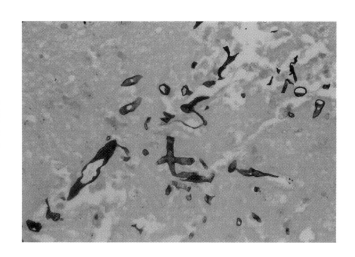

**14-48 *Rhizopus* spp. Lactophenol cotton blue preparation (×80).** The members of the genus *Rhizopus* are characterized by the presence of sporangiophores that grow opposite the rhizoids along the stolon. The columella is round or slightly elongated, and the apophysis is not obvious.

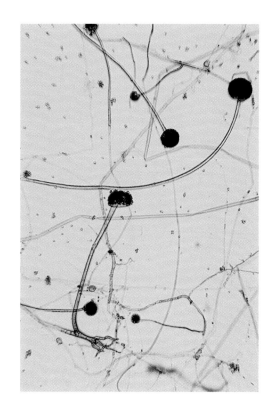

# Subcutaneous Mycoses

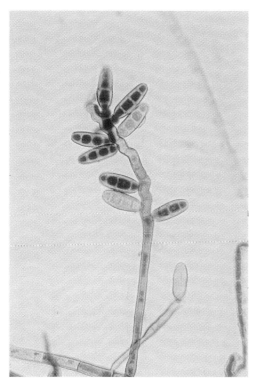

**14-49  Lactophenol cotton blue preparation of *Bipolaris* spp. (×550).** The conidia of *Bipolaris* spp. are fusiform, approximately 10 × 20 μm in size, rounded at both ends, with the central cells similar in size and color to the distal ones, 3 to 5 light pseudoseptae, and a nonprotuberant hilum. The hilum is a "scar" at the point of attachment of a conidium to the conidiophore. The conidiophores bend at each point where conidia are formed, giving a zigzag appearance. The hyphae are septate.

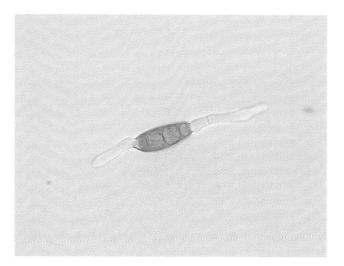

**14-50  *Bipolaris* spp. Germ tube preparation (×575).** *Bipolaris* spp. typically display orientation of the germ tubes along the axis of the conidium. This characteristic can be used to differentiate these organisms from members of the genus *Drechslera*, which form germ tubes perpendicular to the conidial axis. Members of the genus *Exserohilum* also form germ tubes along the axis of the conidium. However, the size and structure of the conidium is significantly different.

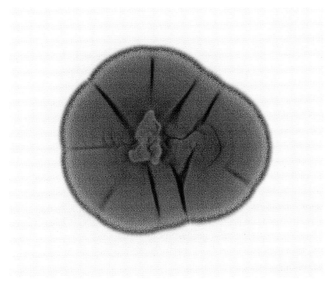

**14-51  Colony of *Cladosporium carrionii* growing on Sabouraud's dextrose agar.** The colonies of *C. carrionii* are slow growers, with a flat or slightly raised center, and a velvety gray or green-black color.

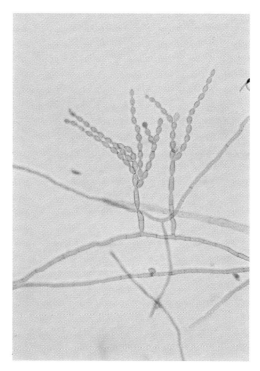

**14-52  *Cladosporium carrionii* preparation stained with lactophenol cotton blue (×550).** The hyphae are dark, septated, and have branches. The conidiophores are elongated and produce chains of ellipsoid, smooth-walled conidia that measure approximately 2 × 5 μm in size. The conidia have a characteristic dark area at the ends called a disjunctor. The conidia closest to the conidiophore may have a "shield" shape.

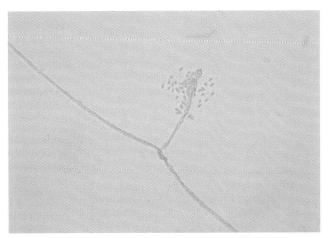

**14-53 *Exophiala (Wangiella) dermatitidis.* Lactophenol cotton blue preparation (×500).** In new cultures, oval and round budding yeastlike cells are formed. Subsequently, these cells produce septate hyphae with flask-shaped to cylindrical phialides. The conidia are round or oval, measure approximately 3 × 5 μm, and are found at the tip of the phialide and also along the hyphae. Growth and biochemical characteristics are used to differentiate these organisms from *Exophiala jeanselmei* and *Phaeoannellomyces werneckii.*

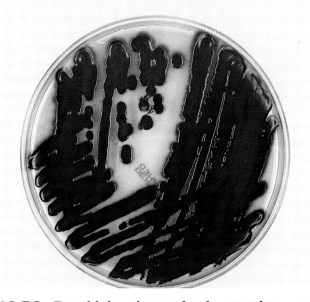

**14-54 *Exophiala jeanselmei* growing on Sabouraud's dextrose agar.** The colonies are brown or green-black, moist, and glistening. With age they become covered with velvety-grayish hyphae. The reverse is black.

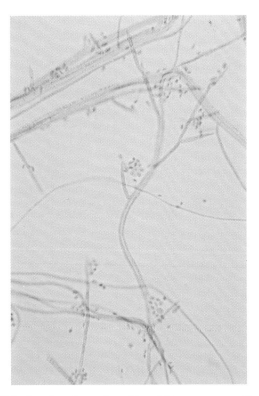

**14-55 Lactophenol cotton blue preparation of *Exophiala jeanselmei* (×500).** The conidiophores are elongated, tubular, and with a tapered, narrow end. The conidia of *E. jeanselmei* are smooth, thin-walled, and ellipsoid, measuring 2 × 3 μm, and can gather in clusters around the conidiophores and at points along the septate hyphae.

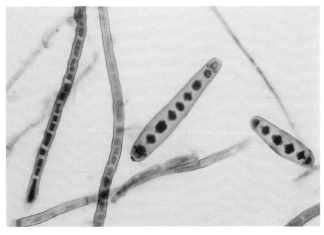

**14-56 Lactophenol cotton blue preparation of *Exserohilum* spp. (×500).** The conidia are fusiform, measure approximately 100 × 15 μm, have a prominent truncated hilum, seven to eleven septa, and the septum next to the hilum is often darkly stained. The conidiophores are elongated and bend at the point of attachment of the conidia (geniculate), giving a zigzag formation. The hyphae are septate and dark.

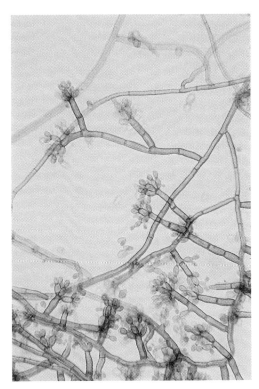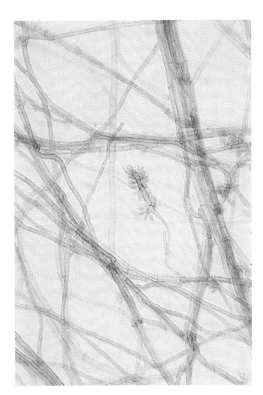

**14-57, 58** *Fonsecaea pedrosoi* **stained with lactophenol cotton blue (×550).** The hyphae of *F. pedrosoi* are septate, branched, and have a dark brown pigment. Three types of conidial formation may be observed. The *Phialophora* type (see *Phialophora* sp.), the *Cladosporium* type, and the *Rhinocladiella* type. In the *Cladosporium* type (Figure 14-57) the conidiophores give rise to large shield-shaped cells that produce branching chains of oval conidia with dark scars in the hila. In the *Rhinocladiella* type of conidiation (Figure 14-58), the conidiophores, arising terminally or laterally on hyphae, have denticles that produce ovoid or elongated conidia along the sides or the tips.

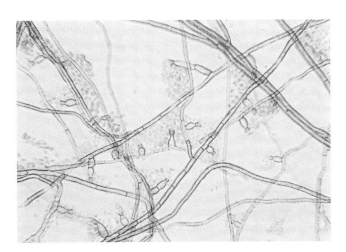

**14-59** *Phialophora verrucosa* **stained with lactophenol cotton blue (×500).** This microorganism has typical vase- or flask-shaped or elliptical phialides, or conidiophores, with wide, flared, pigmented collarettes. The conidia are round or ellipsoid, hyaline, and measure approximately 2 × 4 μm. Hyphae are septate, brown, and branched.

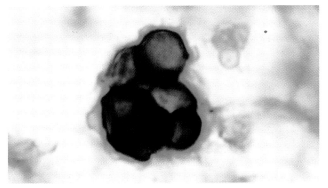

**14-60 Gomori's methenamine silver stain of chromoblastomycosis (×1250).** Skin lesion from a patient with chromoblastomycosis. Thick-walled dark brown cells (called *sclerotic bodies* and the hallmark of chromoblastomycosis) that divide by septation can be observed. The following microorganisms are associated with chromoblastomycosis: *Botryomyces caespitosus, Cladosporium carrionii, Fonsecaea pedrosoi, Fonsecaea compacta, Phialophora verrucosa,* and *Rhinocladiella aquaspersa.*

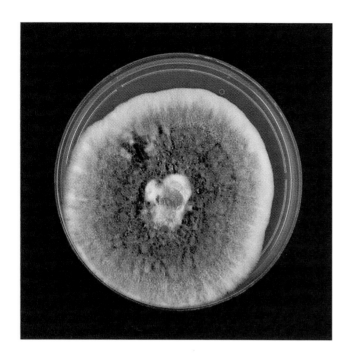

**14-61 Colony of *Pseudallescheria boydii* on Sabouraud's dextrose agar.** The colonies of *P. boydii* have a cottony surface that is white to gray-brown in color and gets darker with the age of the culture. The reverse is also white, turning brown with age.

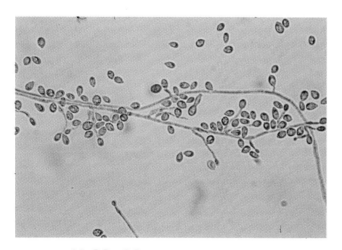 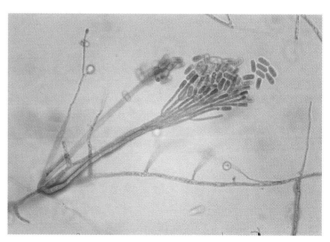

**14-62, 63 Lactophenol cotton blue stain of *Scedosporium apiospermum* and *Graphium* conidia, asexual states of *Pseudallescheria boydii* (sexual state) (×500).** The *Scedosporium* type of conidia of *P. boydii* (Figure 14-62) may rise directly from the septate hyphae or from the tip of coniophores, appear truncated at the base, and sometimes resemble the conidia of *Blastomyces dermatitidis*. The hyphae are long and slender, branch at acute angles and thus may resemble aspergilli. As shown, the coremia or synnemata (conidial structures) of the *Graphium* state of *P. boydii* (Figure 14-63) have terminal hyaline conidia, club-shaped or cylindrical, approximately 6 × 3μm. In the sexual state (P. boydii) large, 50–200 μm in diameter, round, brown cleistothecia are found containing ascospores (not shown).

**14-64 Lactophenol cotton blue preparation of _Scedosporium prolificans_ (×1250).** In the annellation type of conidiation, the conidia are extruded from the tapered tip of the conidiophore, which bears a ring scar for each conidium. The conidiophores, or annellides, are short and do not branch. The conidiogenous cells are flask-shaped, with annellation and terminal conidia. The conidia are ovoid to pyriform (pear-shaped), truncated at the base, with a smooth and thin wall, approximately 3 × 10 μm.

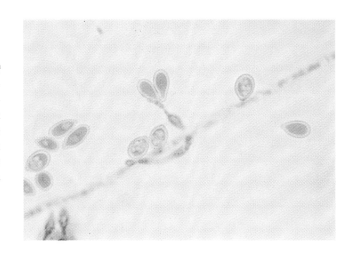

**14-65 Colony of _Sporothrix schenckii_ growing on potato dextrose agar.** At 25°C these colonies grow slowly, are moist, and have a wrinkled surface. The color of the surface initially is white-tan and turns dark brown or black with age. At 37°C the colonies on brain heart infusion agar (BHI) are cream-tan, smooth, and yeastlike (not shown).

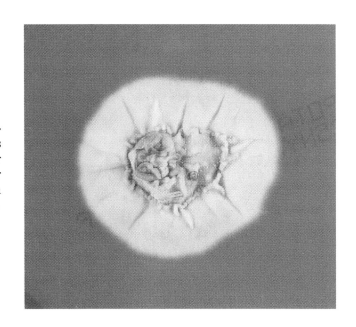

**14-66 Lactophenol cotton blue stained preparation of _S. schenckii_ (×500).** Growth at 25°C produces round, oval, and pear-shaped conidia that measure 2 × 5 μm and are attached to both sides of the septate hyphae by short and thin denticles. Clusters of conidia can also be observed in a "daisy" pattern attached by denticles to conidiophores. At 37°C, oval or fusiform budding cells ("cigarlike") can be observed (not shown).

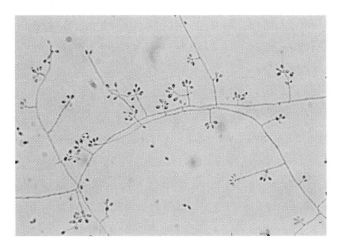

## Superficial Mycoses

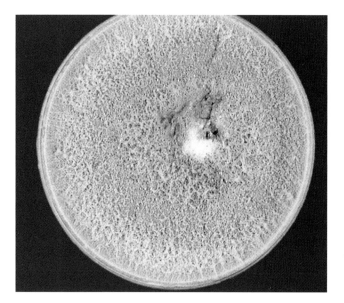

**14-67**  *Epidermophyton floccosum* **on Sabouraud's dextrose agar.** Colonies of *E. floccosum* grow slowly at 25°C and often appear white to tan, although darker colors including olive and khaki can appear with age. The surface is fluffy and powdery and can be flat or radially folded. The reverse side may have an orange-brown pigmentation.

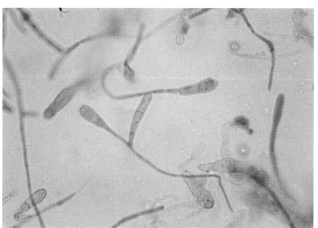

**14-68  Preparation of *E. floccosum* stained with lactophenol cotton blue (×500).** *E. floccosum* have club-shaped, smooth, thin-walled macroconidia that usually grow in clusters directly from the septate hyphae. The macroconidia have less than five septa and measure 20 to 40 by 5 to 8 μm. Chlamydospores, both terminal and intercalary, can be observed in old cultures.

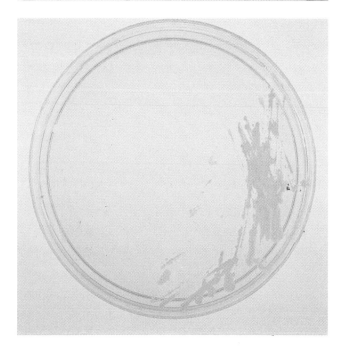

**14-69  Colonies of *Malassezia furfur* growing on Sabouraud's dextrose agar.** Olive oil was added to the right side of the plate. As shown in this figure, the colonies are only growing on the right side of the plate because of the growth requirement of long-chain fatty acids, provided by the olive oil. The colonies grow better at 37°C and are yellow-tan, smooth, and dry.

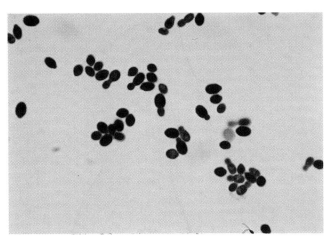

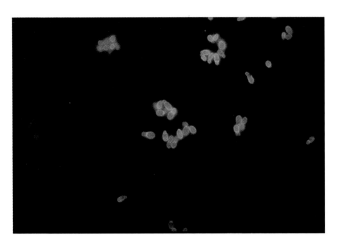

**14-70, 71 Gram stain (14-70; ×1250) and calcofluor white (14-71; ×625) preparations of *Malassezia furfur*.** These yeastlike cells are actually phialides that have a spherical or ellipsoid shape and measure approximately 3 × 5 μm. The cells are round at one end and cut off at the other end, with an indistinct collarette, where the budlike structure forms singly on a broad base. In the calcofluor white fluorescence stain, the typical "bowling-pin" morphology can be clearly observed.

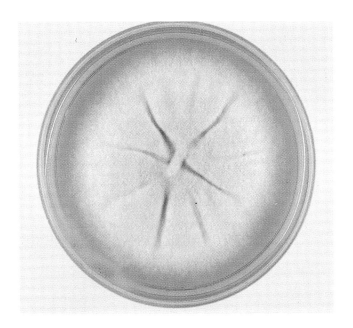

**14-72 *Microsporum audouinii* colony on Sabouraud's dextrose agar.** The colonies of *M. audouinii* are usually white to tan, flat, and have a suedelike surface. The underside is frequently yellow-red-brown.

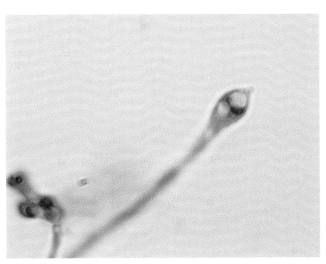

**14-73 *Microsporum audouinii* stained with lactophenol cotton blue (×1800).** Cultures of *M. audouinii* are often sterile. The hyphae are septate with intercalary and terminal chlamydospores. On high magnification, the terminal chlamydospores can be shown to have a pointed end.

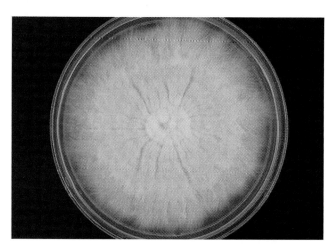
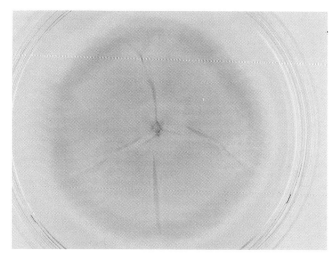

**14-74, 75** *Microsporum canis* **var.** *canis* **colony growing on Sabouraud's dextrose agar.** *M. canis* grows rapidly at 25°C, producing colonies that are usually white-tan with a yellow-green lemon color at the periphery (Figure 14-74). The surface of the colony often has a radiate woolly appearance. The reverse side of the colonies is frequently golden yellow or brown (Figure 14-75).

**14-76 Lactophenol cotton blue preparation of** *Microsporum canis* **var.** *canis* **(×625).** The macroconidia of *M. canis* are spindle or fusiform in shape with a thick irregular rough wall containing between 5 to 15 cells. They measure 5 to 20 by 10 to 100 μm, and characteristically have a knoblike end. The hyphae are septate.

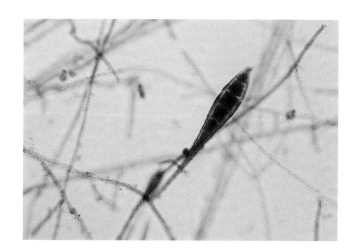

**14-77** *Microsporum gypseum* **colonies on Sabouraud's dextrose agar.** The colonies of *M. gypseum* have a white-tan surface, a white, starburstlike border, and a suedelike appearance. Areas with red-brown color are common on the reverse side. The colonies grow rapidly.

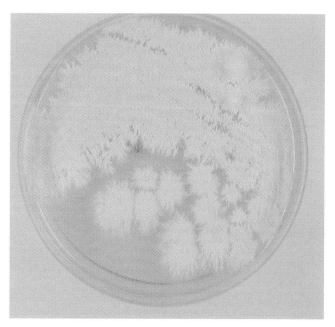

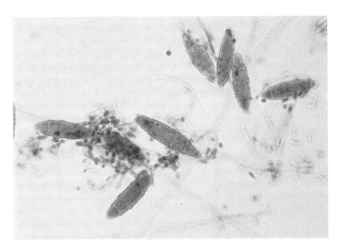

**14-78 *Microsporum gypseum* stained with lactophenol cotton blue (×625).** The macroconidia of *M. gypseum* have an ellipsoidal to fusiform shape with a thin irregular wall, contain four to six cells, and measure 7 to 15 by 30 to 60 μm. The site of attachment to the hyphae is usually flattened, while the distal end is more rounded. The hyphae are septate and the microconidia have a clavate or club shape, but this characteristic is not helpful for differentiation from other fungi that produce similar structures.

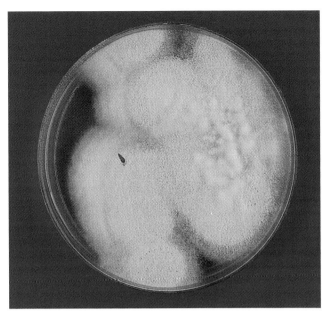

**14-79 Colony of *Trichophyton mentagrophytes* growing on Sabouraud's dextrose agar.** The colonies grow well at 25°C and are usually cream-tan in color, although they may turn darker with age. The surface of the colony appears fluffy and powdery. The reverse of the colony may have a color ranging from tan to brown and dark red.

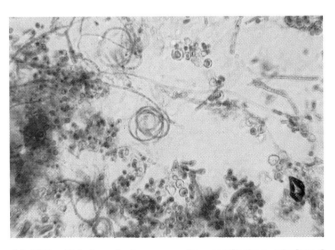

**14-80 *Trichophyton mentagrophytes* stained with lactophenol cotton blue (×500).** This fungus typically displays spherical or pyriform microconidia growing singly or in clusters on branched conidiophores. In addition, there are often characteristic septate spiral or coiled hyphae. Cigar-shaped macroconidia with three to six cells and measuring 7 × 40 μm can sometimes be found (not shown).

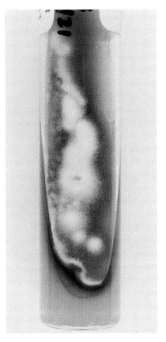

**14-81 *Trichophyton rubrum* on Sabouraud's dextrose agar slant.** White, velvety, or fluffy colonies of *T. rubrum* grown at 25°C. Note the wine-red pigment produced by this organism. Pigments ranging from yellow to orange to red can be observed in different isolates of *T. rubrum*. This type of pigment, however, is not unique to *T. rubrum*. Other dermatophytes, including *T. ajelloi* and *T. mentagrophytes*, can produce red-orange pigments.

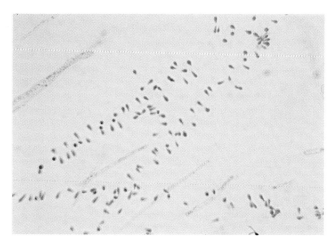

**14-82** *Trichophyton rubrum* **stained with lactophenol cotton blue (×500).** *T. rubrum* has septate hyphae with lateral, tear-shaped microconidia that measure 3 × 4 μm. The macroconidia are long with thin parallel walls and two to eight cells (not shown). Microconidia may form directly from the macroconidia.

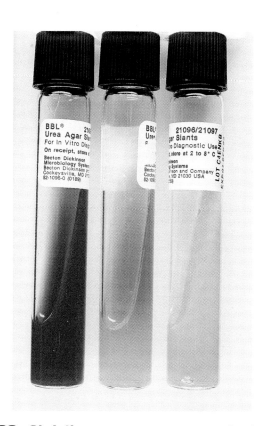

**14-83 Christiansen urea agar slant for demonstrating urease production by *Trichophyton mentagrophytes* and *Trichophyton rubrum*.** The tube on the left side of the image has been inoculated with *T. mentagrophytes*, and the two on the right with *T. rubrum*. The tubes have been incubated for 3, 7, and 3 days, respectively. Note that the *T. mentagrophytes* yields a positive test after 3 days, while the *T. rubrum* is only weakly positive at 7 days.

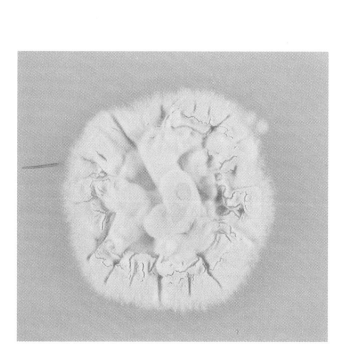

**14-84 Colony of *Trichophyton schoenleinii* growing on Sabouraud's dextrose agar.** Young cultures of *T. schoenleinii* have a waxy appearance with a tan to brown color and honeycomblike thallus (mat of hyphae). This microorganism grows slowly, and with age the colonies become irregular with folded surfaces, as shown in this figure.

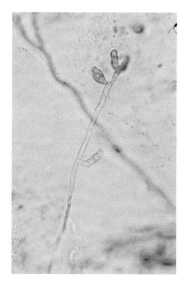

**14-85** *Trichophyton schoenleinii* **stained with lactophenol cotton blue (×500).** The hyphal ends are swollen, giving a "nailhead" morphology, and as a result of branching, often give the appearance of "favic chandeliers" or "antlerlike" hyphae. Macroconidia and microconidia are rare, although chlamydospores are frequently observed.

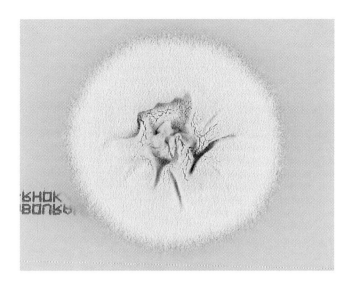
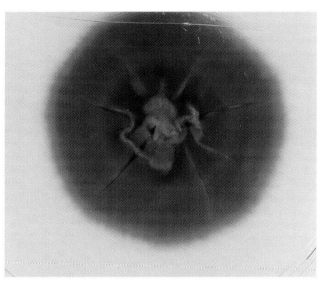

**14-86, 87** *Trichophyton tonsurans* **colony on Sabouraud's dextrose agar.** *T. tonsurans* grows slowly at 25°C on Sabouraud's dextrose agar. The colonies can display a wide variety of colors ranging from white, creamy, yellow, tan, and pink. The colonies can be flat or raised with a velvety or powdery appearance. Note rugae (ruglike folds) cutting across the colony (Figure 14-86). The underside of the colony can range from yellow-brown to red-brown color (Figure 14-87).

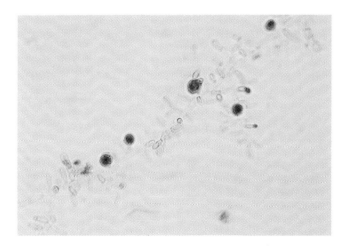
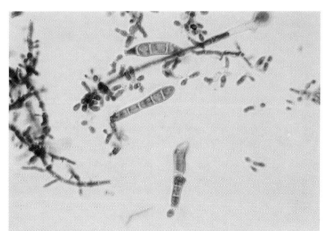

**14-88, 89** *Trichophyton tonsurans.* **Lactophenol cotton blue preparation (×500).** The septate hyphae have microconidia that may vary significantly in size and shape. Some of them are round or oval with a ballooned appearance, and others are clavate and pear-shaped. The microconidia are attached to branched conidiophores by a short stalk (Figure 14-88). Macroconidia are smooth, thin-walled, irregular, and clavate (Figure 14-89), although frequently they cannot be observed. Intercalary and terminal chlamydospores are common.

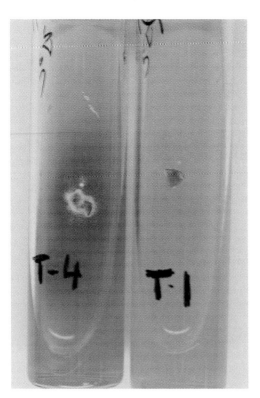

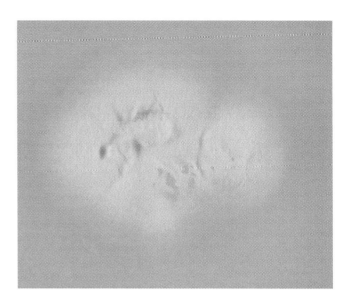

**14-91** *Trichophyton verrucosum* on Sabouraud's dextrose agar. This microorganism has slow-growing colonies with a white, creamy color. The surface is velvety, and the center may be raised.

**14-90 Nutritional test for** *Trichophyton ton-surans.* For this test, the microorganism is grown on vitamin-free casein agar (T1), and on casein agar with thiamine added (T4). As shown in this figure, *T. tonsurans* requires thiamine for growth.

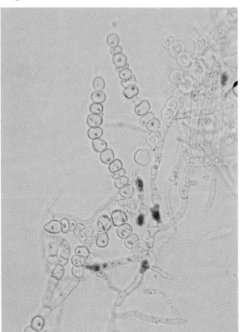

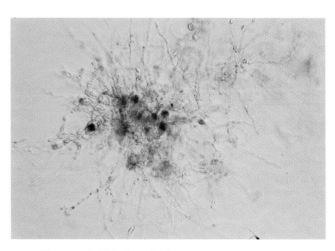

**14-92, 93 Lactophenol cotton blue preparations of** *Trichophyton verrucosum* **(Figure 14-92, ×550; Figure 14-93, ×225).** On Sabouraud's dextrose agar at 37°C, *T. verrucosum* produces many chlamydospores that are sometimes referred to as "chains of pearls" (Figure 14-92). Occasionally "antlerlike" branches at the ends of the hyphae can be observed, but they are rare compared with those of *T. schoenleinii.* On enriched media with thiamine, small, delicate, single microconidia, and long thin macroconidia shaped like a rat's tail can be found (not shown). In some preparations, hyphae produce terminal vesicles (Figure 14-93).

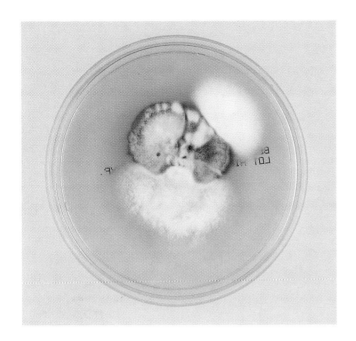

**14-94 Colonies of *Trichophyton violaceum* on Sabouraud's dextrose agar.** *T. violaceum* produces a waxy, irregular shaped, raised colony with areas that have a dark violet color and others that are white. Occasionally, isolates produce only white-tan colonies. The undersurface is purple. In general, this microorganism is a slow grower.

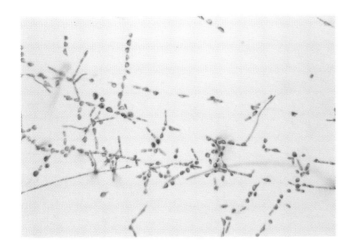

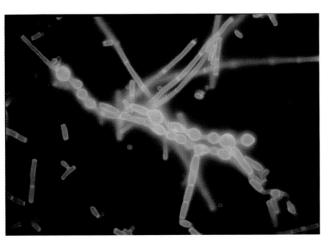

**14-95, 96 Lactophenol cotton blue (14-95; [×225]), and calcofluor white (14-96; [×625]) preparations of *Trichophyton violaceum*.** These figures demonstrate the large, branched, irregular shaped hyphae containing numerous intercalated chlamydoconidia. Macroconidia and microconidia are rarely produced.

# Miscellaneous Mycoses

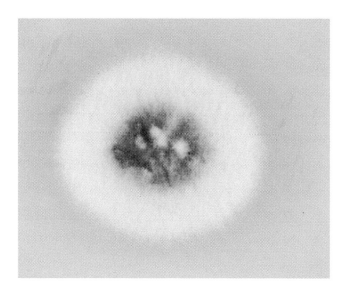

**14-97** *Fusarium* **spp. colony on potato-dextrose agar.** *Fusarium* spp. grow rapidly in culture, and on potato-dextrose agar the colonies are cottonlike, usually white, turning pink-violet or brown at the center with age.

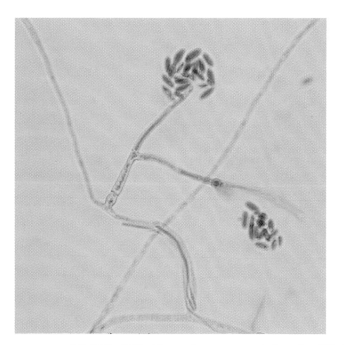

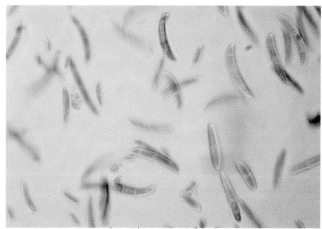

**14-98, 99** *Fusarium* **spp. stained with lactophenol cotton blue (Figure 14-98, ×700; Figure 14-99, ×500).** Typical *Fusarium* spp. microconidia with a fusiform or oval shape extending from delicate lateral phialides (Figure 14-98). The macroconidia of *Fusarium* spp. are produced on conidiophores after 4 to 7 days. The macroconidia are fusiform, usually curved, giving the appearance of a sickle, and have three to five septae (Figure 14-99).

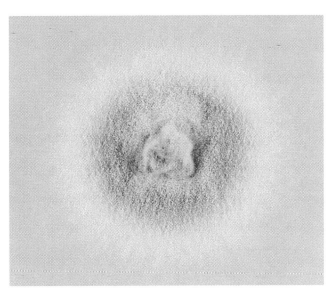

**14-100 Colony of *Paecilomyces variotti* on Sabouraud's dextrose agar.** This organism is a fast grower that produces flat colonies with a tan-brown color and a powdery or suedelike surface.

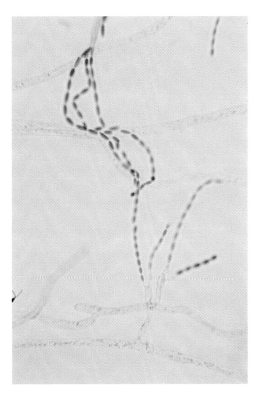

**14-101 Lactophenol cotton blue preparation of *Paecilomyces variotti* (×550).** The phialides, or sterigmata, bend away from the axis of the conidiophore, are elongated and tapered, and thus they are called "ten pins." The conidia are elliptical or oblong, measure approximately 2 × 3 μm, and the chains do not branch.

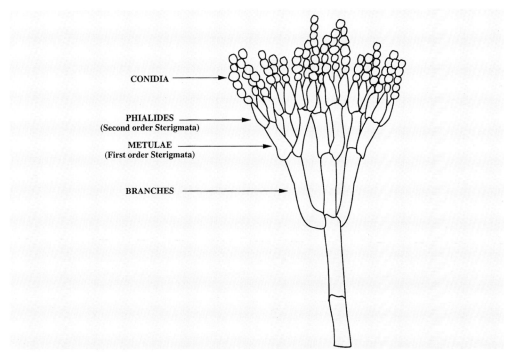

CONIDIA

PHIALIDES
(Second order Sterigmata)

METULAE
(First order Sterigmata)

BRANCHES

**14-102 Diagram of *Penicillium* spp. "brush" or "penicillus."** The septate hyphae have branched and unbranched conidiophores. These form metulae (short, hyphal structures below the phialides) that give rise to flask-shaped phialides. The conidia are round, smooth, or rough and unbranched.

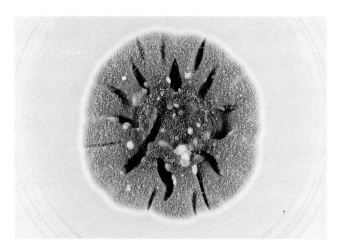

**14-103  Colony of *Penicillium* spp. on Sabouraud's dextrose agar.** The colonies of *Penicillium* spp. usually grow fast and have a powdery white, gray, or green surface color.

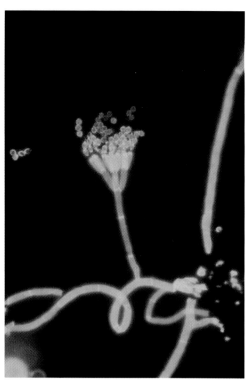

**14-104  *Penicillium* spp. stained with calcofluor white (×250).** Fruiting head of *Penicillium* sp. showing septate mycelia with conidiophores. The conidiophores measure 100 to 250 μm and consist of phialides, or sterigmata, that extend directly from the conidiophore. Alternatively, as in this figure, they originate from metulae, giving a brushlike appearance, also known as a "penicillus." Extending from the tapered tip of the phialides are short, unbranched chains of conidia, measuring 3 × 5 μm, that can be spherical or fusiform and smooth or rough-walled.

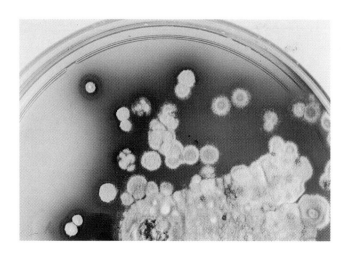

**14-105  Colonies of *Penicillium marneffei* growing on Sabouraud's dextrose agar.** The *P. marneffei* colonies have a white-gray color that turns green with age and produces a characteristic dark red pigment when grown at 25°C.

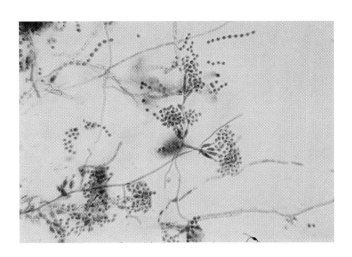 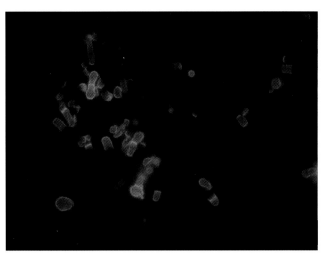

**14-106, 107 Lactophenol cotton blue (14-106; ×500) and calcofluor white (14-107; ×750) preparations of *Penicillium marneffei*.** At 25°C the conidiophores of *P. marneffei* are smooth and have three to five metulae, each of them with several phialides, producing smooth, spherical conidia in chains (Figure 14-106). The conidia measure approximately 3 × 6 μm. At 37°C, oval and elliptical yeastlike cells that measure 3 × 7 μm are produced. The cells replicate by fission and, as shown here, a distinct cross-wall is formed (Figure 14-107).

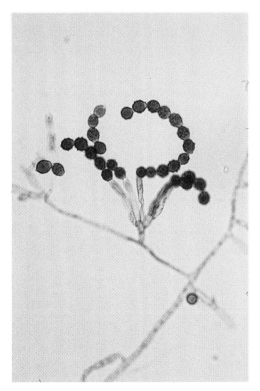

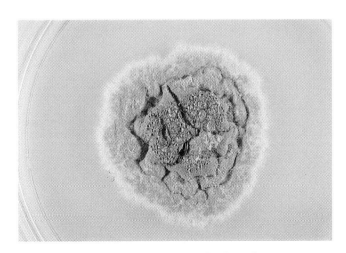

**14-108 Colony of *Scopulariopsis* spp. on Sabouraud's dextrose agar.** This organism grows fast, producing colonies that vary in color from white to tan or brown and black. In most instances however, as in this case, the colony is tan. The surface at first is glabrous (smooth) and with time usually becomes powdery.

**14-109 *Scopulariopsis* spp. stained with lactophenol cotton blue (×550).** This organism typically produces chains of single-celled conidia originating from a conidiogenous annellide. The conidia are round or pyriform, measuring 7 to 8 μm in diameter, with a thick wall that may be smooth or rough, giving the impression of "light globes," and a color that ranges from tan to brown. The hyphae are septate.

# Specimen Preparation and Identification Systems

Colonies of molds isolated in culture can be examined microscopically using several techniques, including the tease mount, the tape mount technique, and the slide culture method. These procedures should always be performed in a laminar flow biosafety cabinet.

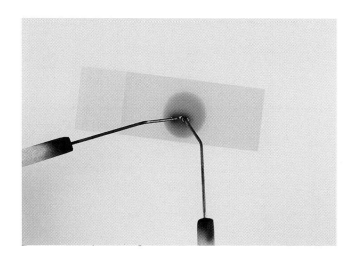

**14-110 Tease mount technique.** For the tease mount, a fragment of the colony is collected using a wire or a loop and transferred to a glass microscope slide. A drop of lactophenol cotton blue is then added, and the specimen is teased using dissecting needles as shown in this figure. The teasing of the specimen needs to be done carefully so that on the one hand, isolated elements can be observed, while at the same time preserving the integrity of the overall structure of the microorganism.

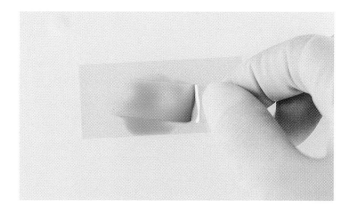

**14-111 Adhesive tape technique.** A piece of transparent adhesive tape is used to collect the specimen by pressing the adhesive side against the surface of the fungal colony. Aerial elements will adhere to the tape, which is subsequently placed on a microscope slide containing a drop of lactophenol cotton blue. This technique is good for preserving the original relationship between spores and aerial hyphae. However, it usually cannot be applied to mold specimens that have few aerial mycelia or to yeast with a moist consistency.

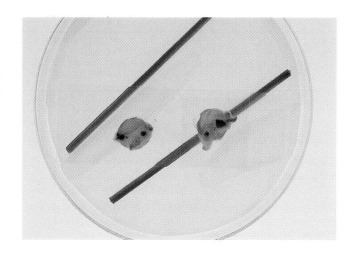

**14-112 Slide culture method.** Two sterile rods are placed at the bottom of a Petri dish on which a sterile glass microscope slide is placed. Blocks or circles of agar are transferred aseptically to the microscope slide. A fragment of the fungal colony to be studied is inoculated onto the sides of the agar, which is coverslipped aseptically and incubated at 25°C. When the colony is mature, the coverslip is removed and both the coverslip and the growth on the slide surface below the agar block are mounted in lactophenol cotton blue and sealed with nail polish or mounting medium.

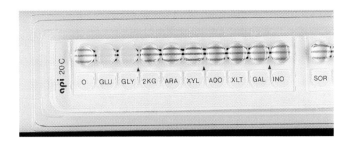

**14-113  API 20C clinical yeast system.** The API 20C system (bioMerieux Vitek, Inc., Hazelwood, Mo.) is a micromethod for the identification of most yeasts and yeastlike microorganisms. Microcupules containing carbohydrate substrates are inoculated with a suspension of the microorganism, and the strip is incubated at 30°C. Once growth occurs, cupules showing turbidity heavier than the 0 control cupule are considered to be positive. The results are converted to a seven-digit biotype, which is matched to the analytical profile index supplied by the manufacturer.

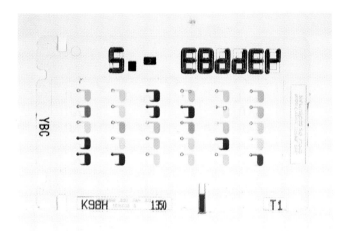

**14-114  VITEK YBC (yeast biochemical card).** The VITEK YBC (bioMerieux Vitek, Inc., Hazelwood, Mo.) card is a component of a semiautomated identification system for yeast and yeastlike organisms. The card contains 30 wells, of which four are negative controls. The biochemical tests include several conventional tests such as carbohydrate assimilation, urea hydrolysis, resistance to cycloheximide, and nitrate reduction. The YBC is incubated at 30°C in the VITEK reader/incubator module, and read at 24 and 48 hours. The automated system provides an identification based on the results of the different reactions.

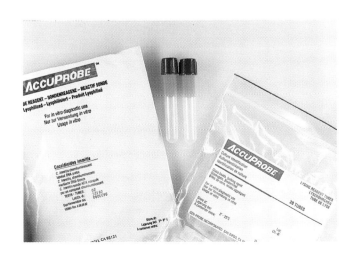

**14-115  DNA probes.** Nucleic acid probes are now available commercially for the identification of *Blastomyces dermatitidis, Coccidioides immitis, Cryptococcus neoformans,* and *Histoplasma capsulatum.* To perform this test, growth from a colony is treated to extract the DNA, which is then hybridized to a probe provided in the kit (Gen-Probe Inc., San Diego, Calif.). One of the main advantages of this system is that the test can be performed before sporulation has occurred.

CHAPTER 15 *Parasitology*

P articularly in areas of poor hygienic practices and sanitation, parasites are still among the major causes of disease and death around the world. Citizens of developed nations often acquire the microorganisms during travel. Direct examination of clinical material is usually the best method for laboratory diagnosis. Careful observation by skilled microbiologists is essential. Serological reagents and tests for some parasites are available commercially and at reference laboratories. This section includes images of protozoa (single-celled microorganisms), followed by helminths (multi-celled microorganisms including worms). Helminths are divided into roundworms, called nematodes; flatworms including flukes, called trematodes; and tapeworms, called cestodes. Average size of the microorganisms is indicated in the legends.

## Protozoans

### Intestinal protozoa: Amebae.

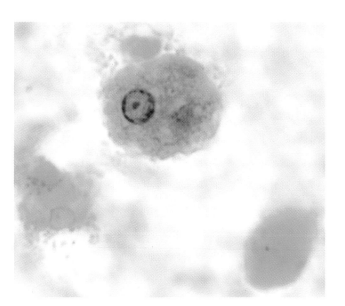

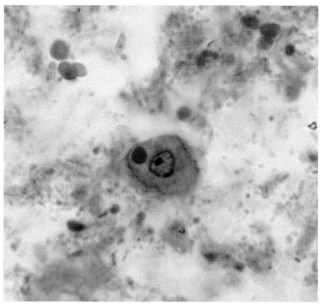

**15-1 *Entamoeba histolytica*. Trophozoites. Feces. Trichrome stain (×2000).** The trophozoites of *E. histolytica* are round and measure from 15 to 30 μm in diameter. With the trichrome stain the cytoplasm stains green-magenta, and the nucleus has a central karyosome. The chromatin has a delicate appearance and is distributed uniformly in the periphery along the nuclear membrane.

**15-2 *Entamoeba histolytica*. Trophozoites. Feces. Trichrome stain (×2000).** This *E. histolytica* trophozoite shows an ingested red blood cell in the cytoplasm. The nuclear structure is still fairly typical although the karyosome is eccentrically located. Ingestion of red blood cells by *E. histolytica* occurs in patients with invasive disease and is considered to be a characteristic that distinguishes this organism from the other species of *Entamoeba*. In addition to red cells, bacteria and cell debris can be found in the phagosomes of this parasite. Macrophages that have ingested cellular material can sometimes be confused with *E. histolytica*.

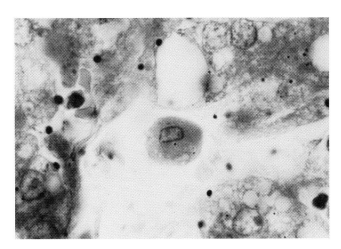

**15-3** *Entamoeba histolytica.* **Trophozoites. Liver. PAS stain (×1250).** Amebic liver abscesses are relatively common complications in cases of invasive disease. The chromatin of this trophozoite is well defined and located along the nuclear membrane. The karyosome is not clearly visible. The morphology of the parasite is usually not well preserved in this type of specimen due to the autolysis of the tissues.

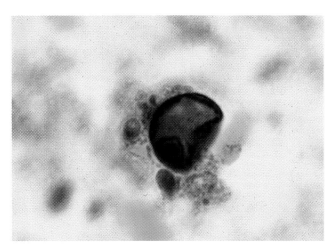

**15-4** *Entamoeba histolytica.* **Cyst. Feces. Trichrome stain (×1500).** Immature cysts of *E. histolytica* typically have a large nucleus that can be laterally displaced by a glycogen vacuole. The karyosome may be, as in this case, large and eccentrically located, although in general, they are small and centrally located. Several chromatoid bodies can be found surrounding the glycogen vacuole. The cysts of *E. histolytica* range in size from 12 to 16 μm.

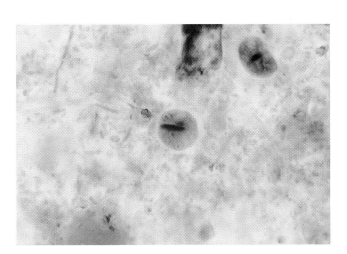

**15-5** *Entamoeba histolytica.* **Cyst. Feces. Trichrome stain (×1250).** Mature cysts of *E. histolytica* have four nuclei while immature cysts contain one or two nuclei. The cysts range in size from 10 to 18 μm and frequently have a diffuse glycogen vacuole, as in this case. Red chromatoid bodies with rounded ends are frequently found. The karyosomes may be slightly eccentrically located, and the peripheral chromatin is fine and evenly distributed.

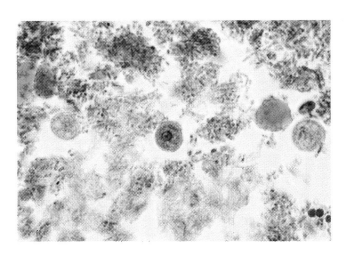

**15-6** *Entamoeba hartmanni.* **Trophozoite. Feces. Trichrome stain (×1250).** The trophozoite of *E. hartmanni* is round or ovoid and measures approximately 7 to 10 μm. With the trichrome stain, the cytoplasm appears green-blue, and the single nucleus demonstrates a karyosome that is usually centrally located, although it can be laterally displaced. The chromatin is peripheral and has a fine appearance. This microorganism does not phagocytize red cells, a characteristic that is useful to distinguish it from *E. histolytica.*

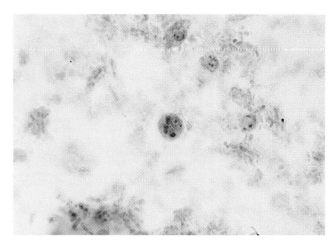

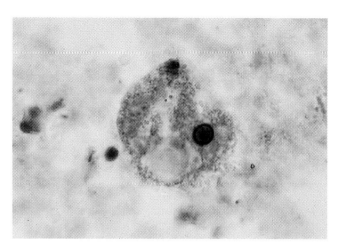

**15-7 *Entamoeba hartmanni*. Cyst. Feces. Trichrome stain (×1250).** The cysts of *E. hartmanni* appear similar to those of *E. histolytica*. Although they are generally smaller in size, 5 to 8 μm, there is a significant amount of overlap, so they are difficult to differentiate. The mature cysts have four nuclei, but the immature cysts with one or two nuclei are more frequently found. The nucleus has a small centrally located karyosome with a uniformly distributed peripheral chromatin. In this particular figure, several typical red-staining chromatoid bodies can be observed.

**15-8 *Entamoeba coli*. Trophozoite. Feces. Trichrome stain (×1250).** The trophozoites of *E. coli* are big, measuring 20 to 25 μm in diameter and are round or ameboid in shape. The single nucleus has a large, eccentrically located karyosome, and the chromatin has a clumpy, irregular appearance that stains green to purple with the trichrome stain. The cytoplasm of this microorganism usually contains bacteria, yeast, and other cell debris. In this figure, a glycogen-like vacuole can be observed in the cytoplasm.

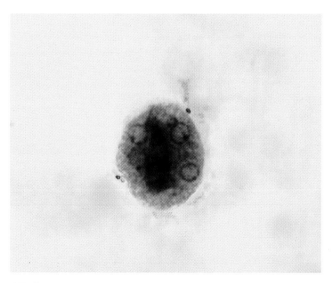

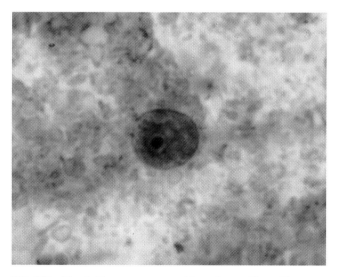

**15-10 *Endolimax nana*. Trophozoite. Feces. Trichrome stain (×2500).** The trophozoites of *E. nana* are small, measuring approximately 8 to 10 μm in diameter. The microorganism is spherical to ameboid in shape and has a cytoplasm that frequently contains granules, vacuoles, and bacteria or other cellular debris. The nucleus is small with a relatively large, red-purple, centrally located karyosome. Trophozoites with irregular karyosomes are frequently found. Typically no marginated chromatin can be observed in the nucleus. This combination of a large karyosome surrounded by a clear halo gives an "owl's-eyelike" appearance to the nucleus of this species.

**15-9 *Entamoeba coli*. Cyst. Feces. Trichrome stain (×2500).** The cysts of this species are large, usually around 15 to 25 μm in diameter, and while the immature cyst has one to two nuclei, the mature stage contains eight nuclei with a distinct, eccentric karyosome. This figure shows four of the eight nuclei in the same plane of focus. The peripheral chromatin is usually coarse, although it may have a smooth appearance. The chromatoid bodies are usually splintered with sharp ends, as shown here.

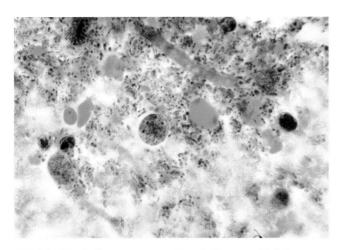

**15-11** *Endolimax nana.* **Cyst. Feces. Trichrome stain (×1250).** The mature cysts measure 7 to 8 μm in diameter, have four nuclei with a prominent karyosome and no peripheral chromatin. No chromatoid bodies are found in the cytoplasm of these microorganisms, although ingested debris and bacteria can be observed.

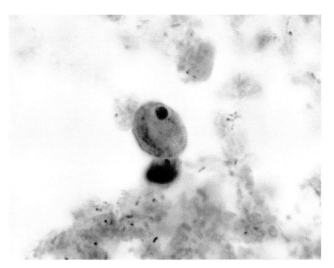

**15-12** *Iodamoeba bütschlii.* **Trophozoite. Feces. Trichrome stain (×2500).** The trophozoites of this species are round or ovoid and measure approximately 12 to 15 μm. The nucleus has a large, reddish, centrally located karyosome with no peripheral chromatin, giving these microorganisms a structural similarity to *E. nana.* Achromatic granules can sometimes be observed between the karyosome and the nuclear membrane.

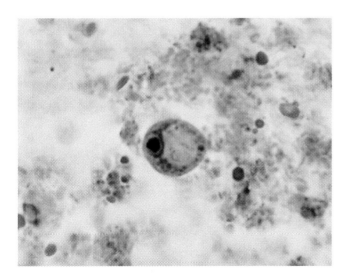

**15-13** *Iodamoeba bütschlii.* **Cyst. Feces. Trichrome stain (×2500).** The cysts of *I. bütschlii* have a single nucleus with a large eccentric karyosome and no peripheral chromatin. Typically the cysts contain large glycogen vacuoles that stain brown with iodine. In this figure, the glycogen is displacing the nucleus to the periphery of the cytoplasm. Cysts range in size from 10 to 15 μm in diameter.

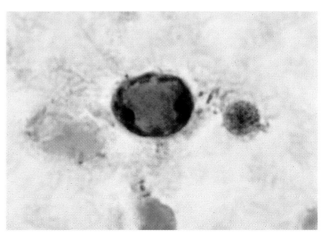

**15-14** *Blastocystis hominis.* **Feces. Trichrome stain (×2000).** This microorganism is oval or spherical and ranges in size from 5 to 35 μm. The central area resembles a vacuole that takes a green color with the trichrome stain. The cytoplasm is located in the periphery and usually contains one nucleus, although two to four can be found. Large granules with a dark red color can also be found in the periphery of the cytoplasm.

## Flagellates and Ciliates

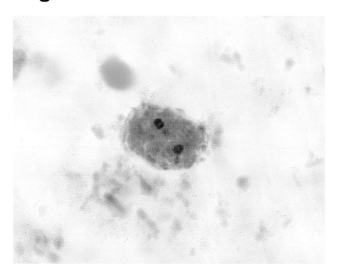

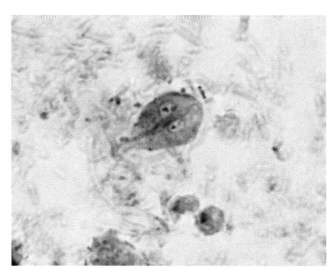

**15-15 *Dientamoeba fragilis*. Trophozoite. Feces. Trichrome stain (×2500).** *D. fragilis* trophozoites resemble ameba and have a spherical or oval shape. They measure 8 to 12 μm, and the cytoplasm frequently contains bacteria, yeast, and other types of debris, giving it a granular appearance. These microorganisms have one or two nuclei with a characteristic karyosome composed of four to eight lobules. No peripheral chromatin can be identified. The small size of *D. fragilis* and the faint structural staining characteristics make its detection difficult. There is no cyst stage in this species.

**15-16 *Giardia lamblia*. Trophozoite. Feces. Trichrome stain (×2500).** The trophozoites of *G. lamblia* have a characteristic pear shape, measuring 10 to 20 μm in length by 10 to 15 μm in diameter. The two nuclei contain a karyosome surrounded by a clear halo and are located one on each side of the axonemes. The karyosomes may appear distinct or may be fragmented. The axonemes extend into eight flagella, four located laterally, two in the ventral region, and two in the caudal section of the microorganism. The dark staining median bodies located below the two nuclei give these microorganisms the appearance of a smiling face. On a lateral view of the microorganisms it is possible to see the sucking disk, used for attachment to the mucosa, that gives the trophozoite the appearance of a "flying saucer" (not shown).

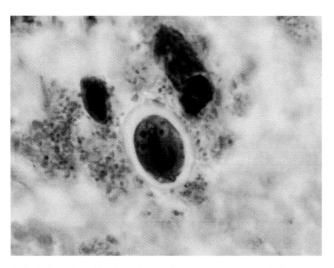

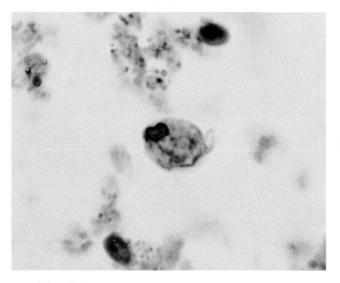

**15-17 *Giardia lamblia*. Cyst. Feces. Trichrome stain (×2000).** The cysts have an oval shape measuring 10 to 15 μm in diameter. The immature cysts have two nuclei that develop into four nuclei in the mature microorganism. These nuclei are usually marginated toward the broader section of the cyst and have prominent karyosomes. Axonemes and fibrils are found in the cytoplasm. As in this figure, retraction of the wall in fixed specimens may give the appearance of a clear halo around the microorganism.

**15-18 *Chilomastix mesnili*. Trophozoite. Feces. Trichrome stain (×2500).** This microorganism is pear-shaped with a pointed end and measures 10 to 25 μm in length by 10 to 15 μm in width. The nucleus in this figure is anteriorly located and has a poorly defined karyosome. The karyosome can be centrally or peripherally placed, and the chromatin is uniformly distributed. A cytostome, a mouthlike structure, may occupy up to one half of the microorganism.

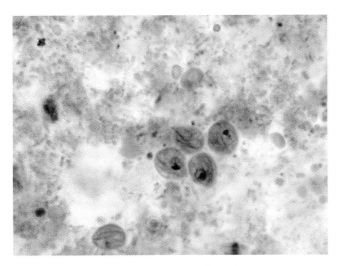

**15-19** *Chilomastix mesnili.* **Cyst. Feces. Trichrome stain. (×1500).** The cyst of this organism has a lemon shape with a hyaline knob at one end. Fibrils present along the side of the cytostome may give the cyst the appearance of an open safety pin. These cysts measure approximately 7 to 9 μm in diameter and are sometimes misidentified as amebas.

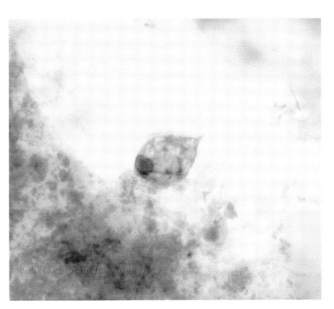

**15-20** *Trichomonas hominis.* **Trophozoite. Feces. Trichrome stain (×2000).** The trophozoites of *T. hominis* have a pyriform shape, measuring 15 to 20 μm in length by 10 to 15 μm in width. The cytoplasm, which may contain granules and a large nucleus, with evenly distributed chromatin, is located at the broad end of the microorganism. An undulating membrane and three to five flagella, four anterior and one posterior, give this microorganism an erratic, brisk movement in wet mount preparations.

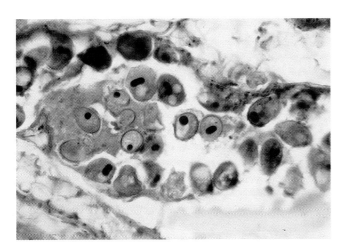

**15-21** *Balantidium coli.* **Trophozoites. Colon biopsy. Hematoxylin and eosin (×225).** Specimen from a human colon containing trophozoites of *B. coli*. The trophozoites are oval with a tapering end, and measure 40 to 50 μm in diameter by 50 to 100 μm in length. The macronucleus is clearly visible in several microorganisms, and the cytostome can also be observed in some of the trophozoites. In viable specimens, the cilia are in constant movement.

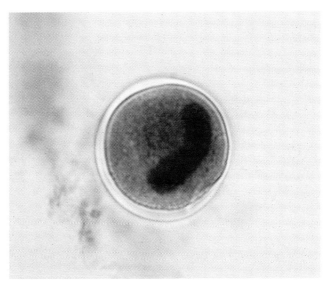

**15-22** *Balantidum coli.* **Cyst. Feces. Carmine stain (×1200).** Cysts are oval to spherical, measuring 50 to 70 μm in diameter. A thick refractive wall can be easily observed. A kidney bean-shaped macronucleus is very distinct in the middle of a fairly uniformly stained cytoplasm in this preparation. An indentation corresponding to the cytostome can be observed on the same side where the macronucleus is located.

# Coccidia and Microsporidia

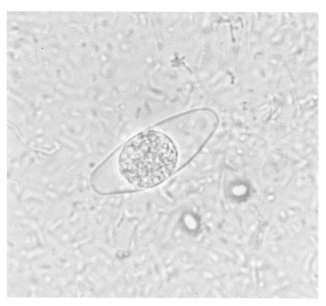

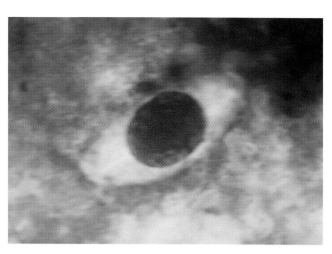

**15-24** *Isospora belli.* **Cyst. Feces. Acid-fast stain (×600).** In acid-fast stained preparations, the body of *I. belli* may appear with an ellipsoid halo around a prominent red-stained spherical sporoblast, as shown here. In other instances, the red stain precipitates along the hyaline wall.

**15-23** *Isospora belli.* **Cyst. Feces. Iodine stain (×1200).** The oocysts are the form more frequently found in the stool; trophozoites are rarely seen. The cyst has the shape of a football measuring 25 to 35 μm in length by 10 to 20 μm in width. The hyaline wall is double-layered, refractive, and is clearly visible in this preparation. In stool specimens, however, the wall may be difficult to observe. A large, centrally located spherical sporoblast is fairly prominent. Mature oocysts contain two sporocysts with four sporozoites each (not shown).

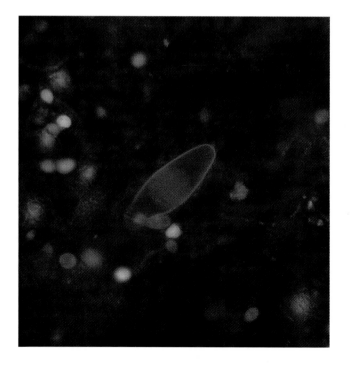

**15-25** *Isospora belli.* **Cyst. Feces. Wet preparation. Autofluorescence (×1250).** One of the properties that can be used to identify *I. belli* in stool preparations is the fact that this microorganism autofluoresces under UV light. The hyaline wall is particularly prominent, and the sporoblasts can also be identified.

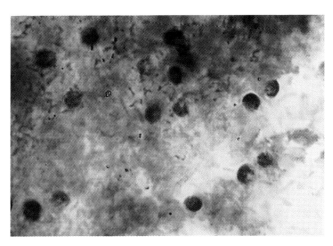
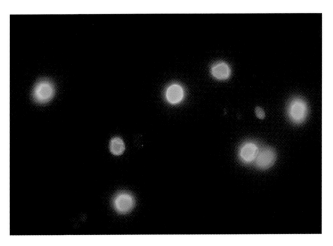

**15-26, 27  *Cryptosporidlum parvum*. Oocysts. Feces. Acid-fast (15-26; ×1250) and fluorescence stain (15-27; ×1250).** In acid-fast stained preparations, the oocysts of *C. parvum* appear round to oval, measuring approximately 4 to 6 μm in diameter. Several black granules can be observed, usually in the periphery of the cyst. Under fluorescence, the wall of the cysts may appear smooth or wrinkled.

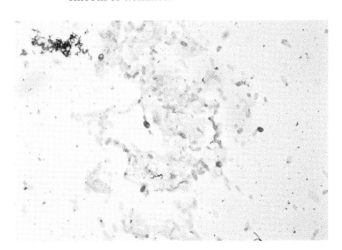
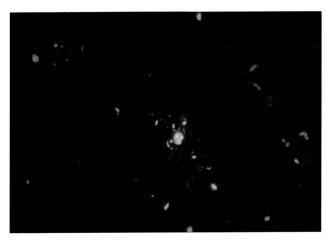

**15-28, 15-29  Microsporidium spp. Feces. Modified trichrome (15-28; ×1250). Calcofluor white stain (15-29; ×1250).** The spores of *Microsporidium* spp. are round or oval and measure 1 to 3 μm. Diagonal bands crossing the cell and corresponding to the polar tubule can sometimes be observed.

## Tissue Protozoa

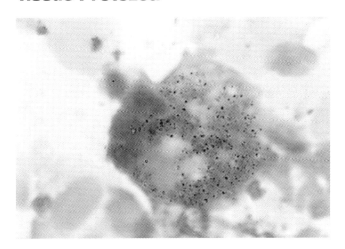

**15-30  *Pneumocystis carinii*. Sputum. Gram stain (×1250).** Both the trophozoite and the cyst form can be observed in respiratory specimens. The microorganisms multiply to form clusters that fill alveolar spaces and block air exchange. The trophozoites are round to oval, measure approximately 5 μm in diameter, and have a nucleus that can be observed with certain stains such as Giemsa.

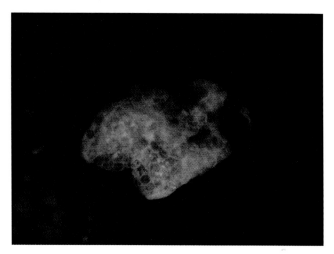

**15-31** *Pneumocystis carinii.* **Bronchoalveolar lavage. Monoclonal antibody stain (×2000).** Often called the "honeycomb" structure, this cluster consists of cysts that measure 5 to 8 μm in size, and when mature, can contain up to eight trophozoites.

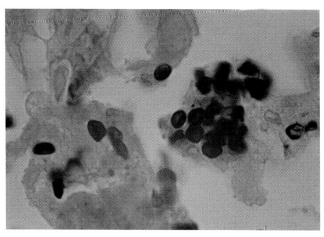

**15-32** *Pneumocystis carinii.* **Lung biopsy. Gomori's methenamine silver stain (×1250).** The cup-shape structure of collapsed cysts is clearly visible in this preparation.

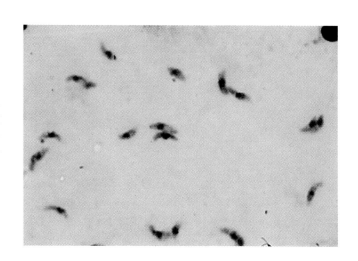

**15-33** *Toxoplasma gondii.* **Trophozoites. Culture. Giemsa stain (×1250).** Trophozoites of *T. gondii* have a crescent shape, measuring 5 to 8 μm in length by 2 to 3 μm in width. The nucleus is relatively large and appears to be centrally located.

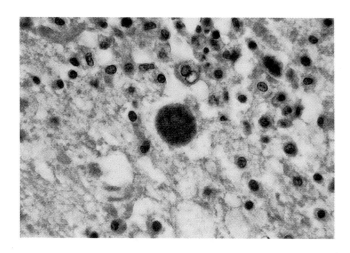

**15-34** *Toxoplasma gondii.* **Cyst. Brain. Hematoxylin and eosin stain (×1250).** Infections with *T. gondii* in humans can result in the formation of cysts in different tissues, including the brain. The cysts can range in size from 5 to 50 μm and may contain up to several hundred microorganisms. The tissue stage of the microorganism is called cystozoite or bradyzoite.

# Malaria and *Babesia* spp.

**15-35–15-51** *Plasmodium falciparum, Plasmodium malariae, Plasmodium ovale,* and *Plasmodium vivax.* **Blood films, thick and thin preparations. Giemsa stain (×1250 except as noted).** Malaria is transmitted to humans by female *Anopheles* spp. mosquitoes. The inoculated sporozoites travel by the bloodstream to the liver where they infect the hepatocytes. After a period of 2 to 3 weeks, they mature into schizonts that release merozoites into the blood and infect the erythrocytes. Inside the red blood cells, the parasite may follow asexual (producing merozoites) or sexual (producing gametocytes) development. The asexual replication cycle repeats itself approximately every 48 hours in the case of *P. falciparum, P. vivax,* and *P. ovale,* and every 72 hours in the case of *P. malariae.* Once inside the red blood cells, merozoites form trophozoites. The trophozoites mature into schizonts that rupture and release merozoites that infect more red blood cells. Gametocytes, on the other hand, represent the sexual stage, which is infectious to mosquitoes. In the mosquitoes, the gametocytes develop into male and female gametes, which undergo fertilization and mature into sporozoites. All stages of the growth cycle of *P. malariae, P. vivax,* and *P. ovale* can be found in the circulating blood. In infections due to *P. falciparum* in the peripheral blood, only ring forms and the gametocytes with the pathognomonic banana, crescent, or half-moon shape are usually observed.

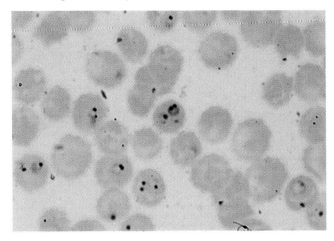

**15-35** *Plasmodium falciparum,* **ring forms.** This species, which causes the most serious disease, often produces heavy parasitemia with double rings, and "headphone" forms. The microorganism does not cause enlargement of the cytoplasm of the parasitized erythrocyte, but it may induce formation of large, purplish Maurer's dots, as seen in the central red blood cell in this preparation.

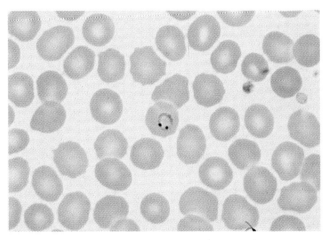

**15-36** *Plasmodium falciparum,* **ring form.** Visible is a "headphone" structure created by two dots of chromatin on the same ring.

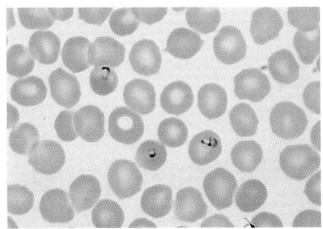

**15-37** *Plasmodium falciparum.* A later trophozoite stage is on the right. This stage is not usually observed on specimens from patients with a *P. falciparum* infection. However, it is frequently found in cases of infection with the other three species of *Plasmodium.*

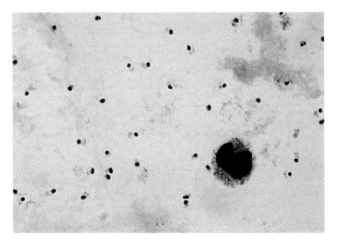

**15-38** *Plasmodium falciparum.* **Thick blood smear.** Multiple ring forms are visible.

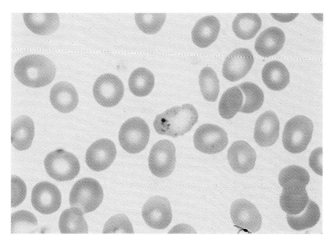

**15-39** *Plasmodium vivax.* The infected red blood cells can be enlarged up to twice their normal size when infected by *P. vivax* or *P. ovale.* Eosinophilic cytoplasmic stippling, called Schüffner's dots, are also present in erythrocytes infected with these two species. This infected red blood cell is enlarged and displays Schüffner's dots.

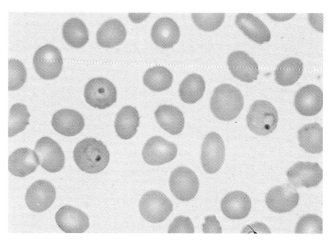

**15-40** *Plasmodium vivax.* Infected cells show fine stippling of Schüffner's dots around the edges and the typical heavy chromatin dot.

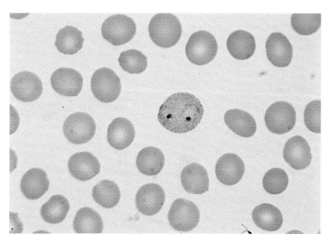

**15-41** *Plasmodium vivax.* Although double ring forms are suggestive of *P. falciparum,* the large cell size and obvious Schüffner's dots help to identify this infection as *P. vivax.*

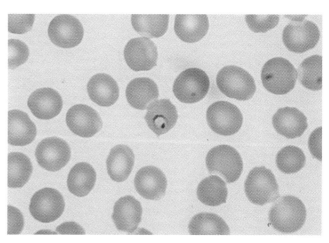

**15-42** *Plasmodium ovale.* The enlarged size and irregular edge of this infected erythrocyte are typical of *P. ovale* infection. Schüffner's dots, often present with *P. ovale* infections, are absent here.

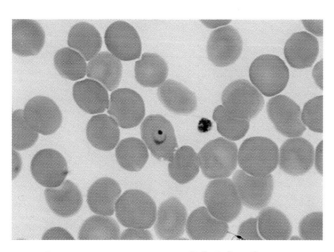

**15-43** *Plasmodium ovale.* Infected erythrocytes may develop a fimbriated edge, shown here.

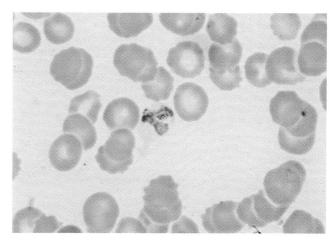

**15-44** *Plasmodium malariae.* Band-form trophozoite, seen almost exclusively in *P. malariae.* Schüffner's dots are absent in infections with this species.

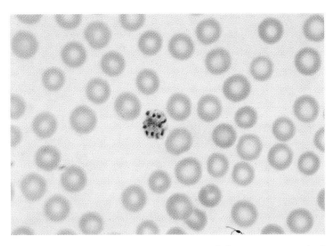

**15-45** *Plasmodium malariae.* Schizonts in a typical rosette formation. The schizonts of this species typically contain six to 10 merozoites. Hemozoin pigment, brown in color, is also visible. The pigment is present in schizonts of all four species but is most prominent in *P. malariae.*

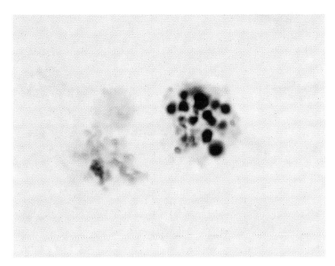

**15-46** *Plasmodium vivax.* **Thick blood smear (×3500).** Mature schizonts of *P. vivax* have on the average 16 merozoites, although the number can range from 12 to 24. The pigment is usually golden-brown and not very prominent.

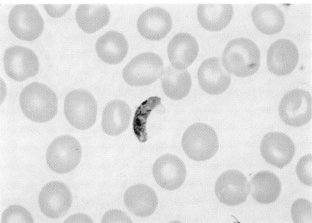

**15-48** *Plasmodium falciparum.* Banana-shaped gametocyte seen only in infections due to this species. Peripheral blood reveals only gametocytes and ring forms in *P. falciparum* infections. At the gametocyte stage, the red cell membrane may be invisible.

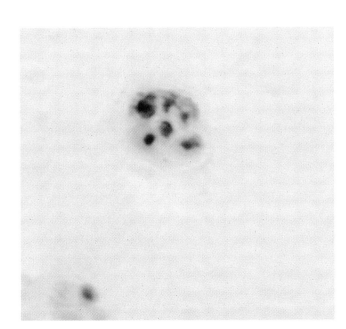

**15-47** *Plasmodium ovale.* **Thick blood smear (×3500).** Although schizonts of this species develop up to 16 merozoites, they can reveal fewer numbers during early stages of development. Hemazoin pigment is most difficult to see in schizonts of this species.

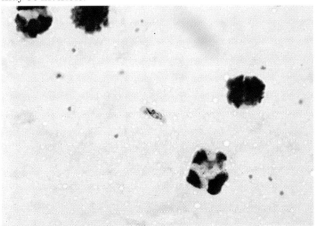

**15-49** *Plasmodium falciparum.* **Thick blood smear.** Crescent-shaped gametocyte displays prominent brown pigment.

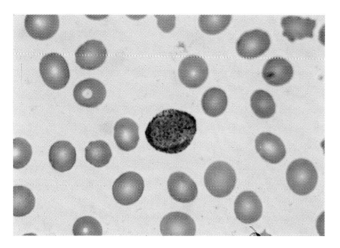
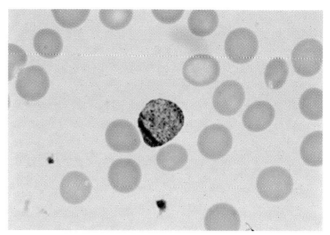

**15-50, 51** *Plasmodium vivax,* **macrogametocytes.** The micro- and macrogametocytes of *P. vivax, P. malariae,* and *P. ovale* are large, oval to round bodies. The chromatin of the macrogametocyte is usually more basophilic than that of the microgametocyte.

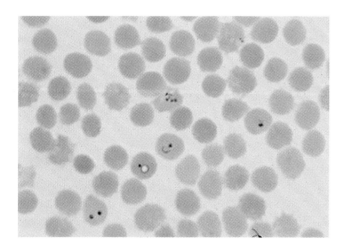
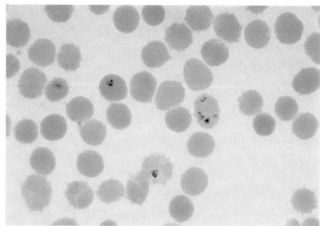

**15-52, 53** *Babesia microti.* **Blood. Giemsa's stain (×1250).** *B. microti* is transmitted in the United States by the tick *Ixodes scapularis,* the same vector that transmits *Borrelia burgdorferi.* The intraerythrocytic form of *Babesia* spp. are round to oval and measure 1 to 5 μm in length. This microorganism reproduces by asexual budding into two to four daughter cells. As shown in these two figures, *B. microti* infects RBCs and produces small, ringlike forms, with a scant amount of cytoplasm and a minute chromatin dot. Some of the RBCs show the characteristic tetrads. In some preparations, these tetrads may appear with a "Maltese cross" configuration. This microorganism should be differentiated from the agent of malaria—in particular, *P. falciparum.* In addition to the presence of the tetrads, in *B. microti* infections, extracellular merozoites can be found, while the brown pigment deposits of hemozoin observed in *Plasmodium* spp. infections are absent.

# Leishmaniasis

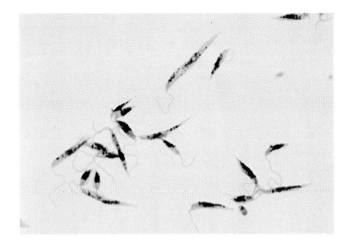

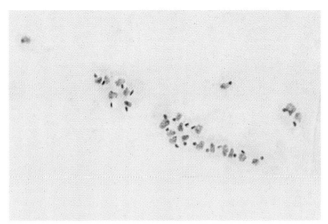

**15-54  *Leishmania* spp. Promastigotes. Culture. Giemsa stain (×1250).** Promastigotes of *Leishmania* spp. are found in the gut of the sandfly where they replicate and subsequently migrate to the proboscis. The vertebrate host is infected at the time of feeding. As shown in this figure, the promastigotes are cigar-shaped, measuring 10 to 12 μm in length, and have a nucleus in the center of the body. The rodlike kinetoplast is located in the anterior part. The flagellum extends from the anterior end, and an undulating membrane can be observed at this stage of development.

**15-55  *Leishmania* spp. Amastigotes. Blood preparation. Giemsa stain (×1250).** The amastigotes of *Leishmania* spp. are oval and measure 4 to 5 μm in length by 2 to 3 μm in diameter. A dark-staining kinetoplast can be observed close to the nuclei in some of the microorganisms. This is the only stage found in humans. This microorganism can be confused with *Histoplasma capsulatum*, *Toxoplasma gondii*, and *Trypanosoma cruzi*.

# Trypanosomiasis

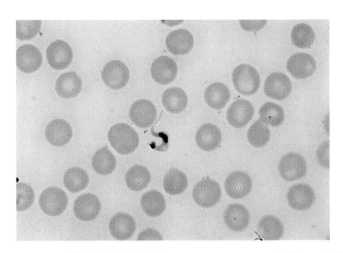

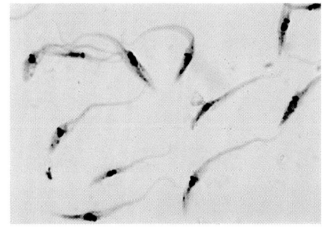

**15-56, 57  *Trypanosoma cruzi*. Blood (15-56) and culture (15-57). Giemsa stain (×1250).** Typical C-shape trypanomastigote of *T. cruzi* (15-56). This microorganism is the cause of the American trypanosomiasis, or Chagas' disease. It measures approximately 15 to 20 μm in length, has a central nucleus, and a conspicuous kinetoplast. The free flagellum measures 5 to 10 μm, and the undulating membrane is not as prominent as the one in the African trypanosomes. Figure 15-57 demonstrates trypanomastigotes of T. cruzi growing in NNN medium.

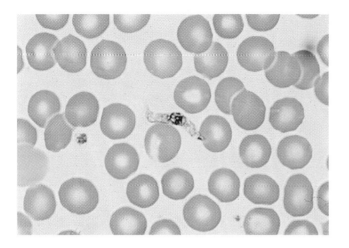

**15-58 *Trypanosoma brucei gambiense*. Mouse blood. Giemsa stain (×1250).** *T. brucei gambiense* and *T. brucei rhodesiense* are the causative agents of African trypanosomiasis, or sleeping sickness. The trypanomastigotes of *T. brucei gambiense* have a nucleus, a kinetoplast located at the blunt posterior end, and an undulating membrane with a flagellum. In general, the trypanomastigotes are spindle-shaped and measure 20 to 30 μm in length.

## Other Protozoa

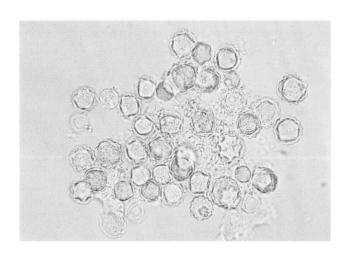

**15-59 *Acanthamoeba* sp. Cyst from agar culture. Wet mount (×500).** The cysts of *Acanthamoeba* sp. are spherical and measure approximately 15 to 18 μm in diameter. Typically the wall has two layers. The outer wall is wrinkled, while the internal wall may be smooth or may appear polygonal or spherical. The trophozoites of *Acanthamoeba* are large, measuring 20 to 40 μm in diameter, and have thin extensions called acanthopodia (not shown). The cytoplasm appears irregular and contains different types of vacuoles. The karyosome is large and centrally located in the nucleus. No peripheral chromatin can be observed in this microorganism.

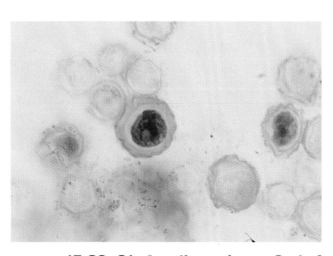
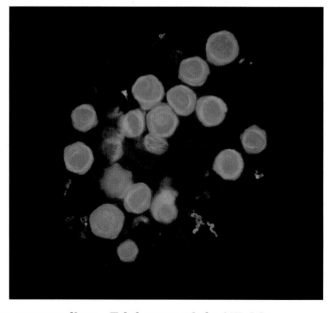

**15-60, 61 *Acanthamoeba* sp. Cysts from agar culture. Trichrome stain (15-60; ×1250). Calcofluor white (15-61; ×500).** With trichrome stain the membrane of *Acanthamoeba* sp. appears green-cyan with the typical wrinkled appearance. The cytoplasm stains red, and the nucleus has a prominent karyosome surrounded by a clear halo. With the calcofluor white stain, the typical wrinkled appearance of the cyst wall is very distinct.

# Nematodes

## Intestinal nematodes

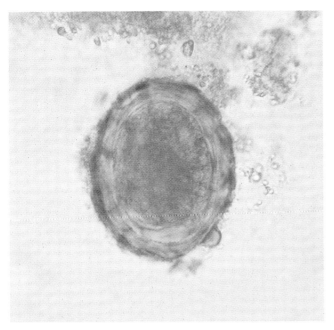

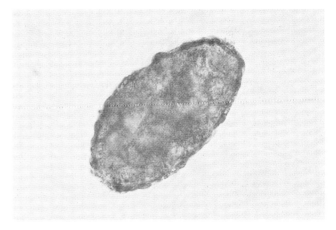

**15-62 *Ascaris lumbricoides*. Fertile egg. Feces. Iodine stain (×900).** The typical fertile *A. lumbricoides* egg is yellow-brown, has a thick, mammillated shell, is oval in shape, and measures approximately 60 × 40 μm. These eggs may lack the external mammillated layer and can be differentiated from hookworm and pinworm eggs by their size and shape.

**15-63 *Ascaris lumbricoides*. Infertile egg. Feces. Iodine stain (×600).** The infertile eggs of *A. lumbricoides* are oval, large (approximately 90 × 45 μm), lack one or more of the shell layers, and the contents have a heterogeneous appearance due to the presence of fat globules and refractive granules.

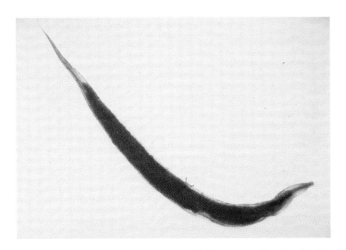

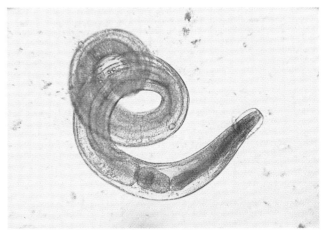

**15-64, 65 *Enterobius vermicularis*. Female (15-64) and male (15-65) adult worm.** The female adult worm of *E. vermicularis* (pinworm) is white and measures from 8 to 15 mm in length by approximately 0.4 mm in width. In contrast, the male adult worm is much smaller, measuring 2 to 3 mm in length by 0.1 to 0.2 mm in width. The dilated cephalic region is similar in both sexes, while the tail is pointed in the females and blunted in the males. Females are more frequently found in cellophane tape preparations than the males. The cephalic inflation of the cuticle and the muscular and bulbous portions of the esophagus separated by a narrow region can be observed in Figure 15-65.

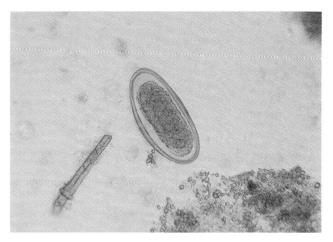

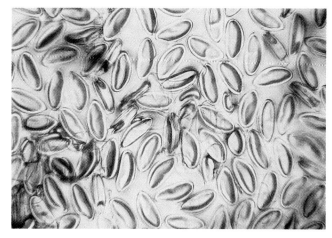

**15-66 *Enterobius vermicularis*. Eggs. Feces. Iodine stain (×600).** Occasionally the eggs of *E. vermicularis* can be found in the feces. The eggs are oval in shape, with one side flattened, and measure in the range of 50 × 25 μm. When the eggs are laid, they are partially embryonated and, as shown in this figure, no larvae can be observed. Eggs reach the infectious stage 5 to 10 hours after they are laid.

**15-67 *Enterobius vermicularis*. Eggs. Cellophane tape preparation (×225).** The females lay eggs at night in the perianal region. Thus, the best time to collect the specimen with cellulose tape is early in the morning. The shell of the eggs is thick and hyaline. In some of the eggs, it is possible to observe the larvae (not shown).

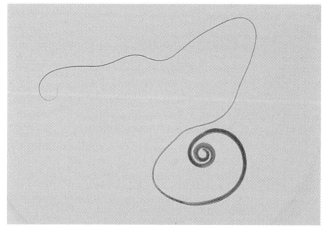

**15-68 *Trichuris trichiura*. Male adult worm (×7.5).** The female worms measure 40 to 50 mm, while the male worms usually range from 35 to 45 mm. In the male, the posterior end is coiled, while in the female it is straight. Both sexes have a whiplike overall shape with a slender anterior end and a thicker, short posterior region.

**15-69 *Trichuris trichiura*. Egg. Feces. Iodine stain (×800).** The morphology of the *T. trichiura* eggs is fairly characteristic. The eggs are oval in shape, measuring 50 × 25 μm, with a thick hyaline wall that has two distinct mucoid condensations, or "plugs," at each end. The eggs are not embryonated in the stools. Embryonated eggs may be found in the soil 2 to 3 weeks after they are passed.

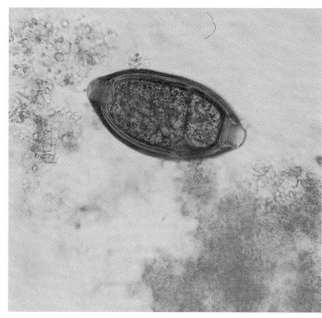

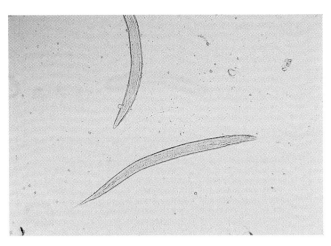
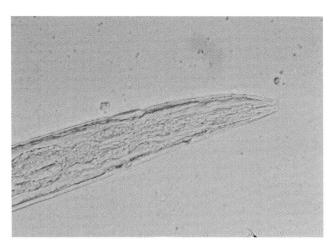

**15-70, 71** *Necator americanus.* **First-stage rhabditiform larvae. Iodine stain (15-70; ×100, and 15-71 ×500).** The first-stage rhabditiform larvae of *Necator americanus* measure approximately 220 to 280 μm in length by 16 to 18 μm in width. The buccal canal (Figure 15-71) is long, while the genital primordium is small and difficult to see.

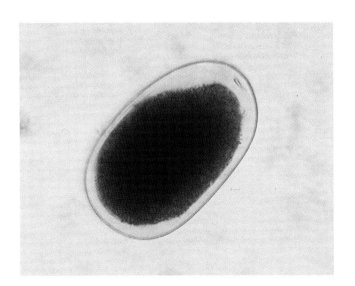

**15-72 Hookworm egg. Feces. Iodine stain (×900).** The eggs produced by *Necator americanus* and by *Ancylostoma duodenale* are indistinguishable. The eggs are oval, large (70 × 40 μm), and have a thin shell. These embryonated eggs have from four to eight cells at the time they are passed in the stool, and they can develop first-stage larvae in a day or two when left at room temperature. This is in contrast to the first-stage larvae of *Strongyloides stercoralis* that are found directly in the feces.

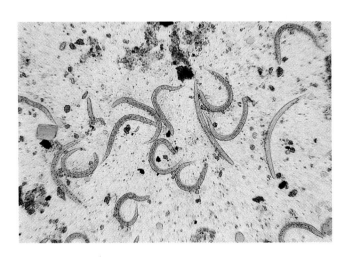

**15-73** *Strongyloides stercoralis.* **First stage rhabditiform larvae. Feces. Iodine stain (×75).** The first-stage larvae are found directly in the feces and are the diagnostic stage of this microorganism. They measure 200 to 400 μm in length by 15 to 20 μm in width. The parasitic adult female measures approximately 2 to 3 mm in length by 30 to 40 μm in diameter. The pointed tail in the female is straight, and eggs can usually be observed in the genital tract. Females are parthenogenetic, and parasitic males do not exist. The male is smaller than the female worm and can be identified by its curved, pointed tail. The parasitic female produces embryonated eggs in the mucosal epithelium of the small intestine. The embryonated egg hatches in the mucosa of the epithelium, and the first-stage larvae migrate to the lumen and are passed in the feces. Subsequently, these larvae mature into the third-stage larvae that are infectious.

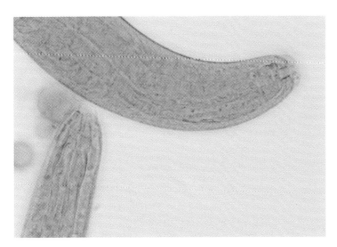
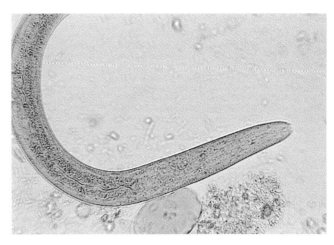

**15-74, 75  *Strongyloides stercoralis*. First-stage rhabditiform larvae. Feces. Iodine stain (15-74, ×1250; 15-75, ×500).** The first stage larvae of *S. stercoralis* have a short buccal canal (as shown here) in contrast to the hookworm larvae that have a long buccal canal. In addition, in the *S. stercoralis* first-stage larvae, the genital primordium is quite apparent (Figure 15-75), while in the hookworm larvae, the genital primordium cannot be seen.

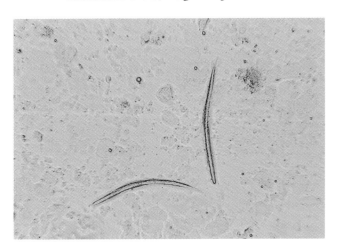
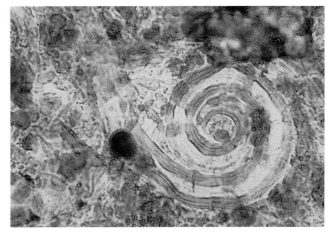

**15-76, 77  *Strongyloides stercoralis*. Filariform larvae. Wet mount (15-76, ×75). Rhabditiform larvae. Sputum. Gram stain (15-77, ×500).** In immunocompromised patients, hyperinfection may result in multiplication of *S. stercoralis* in the intestinal tract, invasion of the wall, and migration of the third stage larvae to all the tissues. In this case the patient had invasion of the lung, and the larvae were observed on a wet mount preparation and on a Gram stain of the sputum. The filariform larva measures 400 to 500 μm in length, the tail is notched (not shown), and the esophagus occupies close to half of the body length.

## Tissue nematodes

**15-78  *Trichinella spiralis*. Larvae, Muscle. Hematoxylin and eosin stain (×225).** The adult female produces larvae in the intestinal mucosa that migrate to the muscle, where they become encapsulated by the host tissues. These larvae measure up to 1 mm by the time they mature, but initially they are approximately 100 μm in length by 5 μm in diameter.

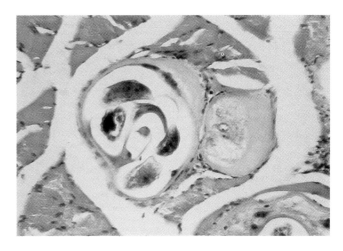

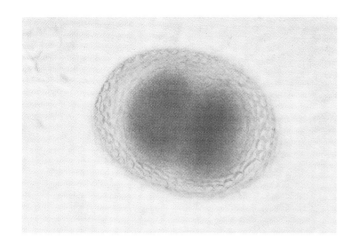
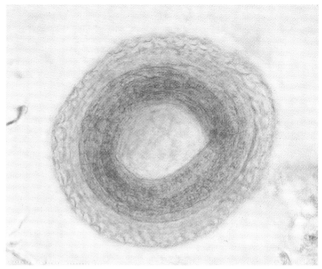

**15-79, 80**  *Toxocara canis.* **Embryonated egg (15-79, ×550) and egg with larvae (15-80, ×700). Dog feces. Iodine stain.** The eggs of *T. canis* are spherical or oval, measuring 85 × 75 μm, with a thick and pitted shell. These eggs are passed in the feces by dogs. Persons coming into contact with these feces, or contaminated soil, can acquire the infection by ingesting the infective eggs. The infection in humans is diagnosed by serology or by identifying the larvae in histological sections.

## Filaria

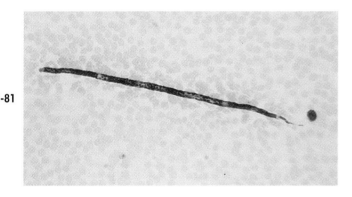
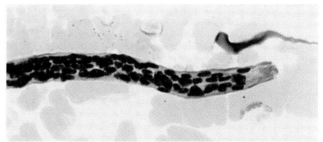
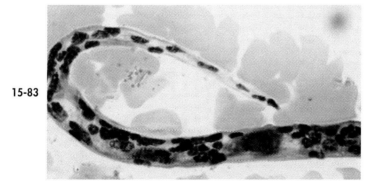

**15-81-15-83**  *Loa loa.* **Microfilariae. Blood, Giemsa stain (15-81, ×600; 15-82 and 15-83, ×1250).** The microfilariae of *L. loa* measure approximately 240 × 7 μm. Although the sheath is not visible on Giemsa stain, a clear halo can sometimes be observed surrounding the microorganism. The cephalic region does not have nuclei (15-82). Typically four to six nuclei at the tip of the tail are spaced evenly and extend to the end (15-83). Deerflies of the genus *Chrysops* transmit the microfilariae, which appear in the blood during the day. The adult microorganism moves through the subcutaneous tissues, producing an inflammatory reaction termed *Calabar,* and can enter the eye and migrate through the conjunctiva. The female adult worms measure 50 to 70 mm by 0.5 mm, while the males are usually half that size.

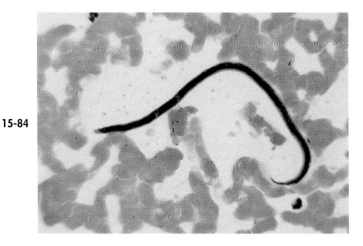

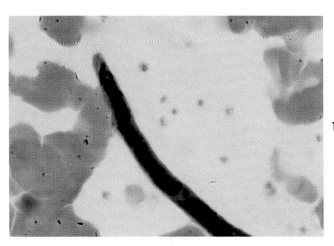

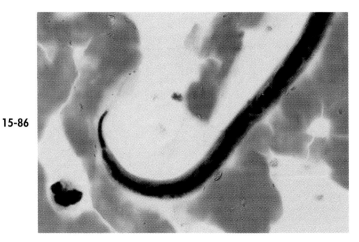

**15-84–15-86** *Wuchereria bancrofti.* **Microfilariae. Blood, Giemsa stain (15-84, ×500; 15-85 and 15-86, ×1250).** The adult worm measures 4 to 10 cm in length and lives in the lymphatics, producing fibrosis and obstruction. The microfilariae are transmitted by several kinds of mosquitoes including *Aedes* spp., *Culex* spp., and *Anopheles* spp. The microfilariae are sheathed and measure approximately 250 μm × 8 μm (Figure 15-84). The cephalic region is round (Figure 15-85), while the tail is pointed (Figure 15-86). Both areas have an end space devoid of nuclei. The microfilariae are found in the lungs during the day while they circulate in the peripheral blood at night.

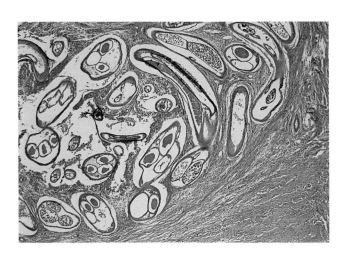

**15-87** *Onchocerca volvulus.* **Tissue section. Hematoxylin and eosin stain (×30).** The microfilariae of *O. volvulus* are produced by the adult female worms and become distributed in the skin. The female blackflies, *Simulium* spp., ingest these larvae when they bite. Following a developmental period of 1 to 2 weeks in the fly, the larvae are again infective to humans when the fly next bites. The adult worms produce nodules in the subcutaneous tissues or in fascial planes. Onchocercal nodules are usually well demarcated by a thick band of connective tissue. Worms from both sexes are embedded in a chronic inflammatory infiltrate containing numerous blood vessels and giant cells. Microfilariae in the surrounding connective tissues produce an inflammatory infiltrate with plasma cells, eosinophils, and lymphocytes.

# Trematodes

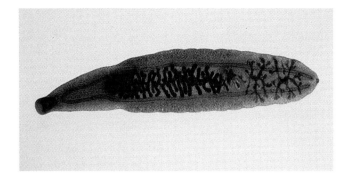

**15-88** *Clonorchis sinensis.* **Adult worm (flukes). Carmine stain (×18).** The adult form of these trematodes lives in the biliary tract of humans. The adult worms measure approximately 10 to 30 mm in length by 2 to 5 mm in width. The microorganism has a ventral sucker and the coiled uterus, ovary, and two branched testes occupy most of the body.

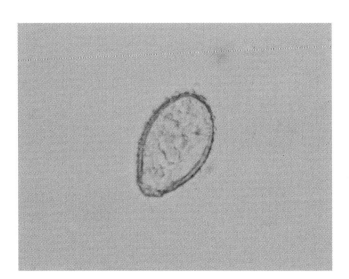

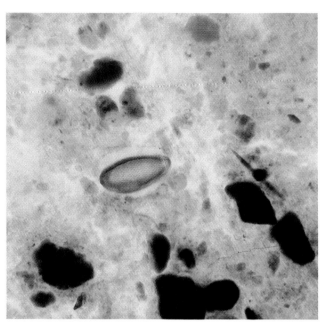

**15-89, 90** *Clonorchis sinensis* **eggs. Iodine (15-89, ×1300) and trichrome stains (15-90, ×800).** The eggs of *C. sinensis* are ovoid and measure approximately 30 × 15 μm. The shell is relatively thick, and there is a well-defined operculum at the narrow end, and a small knob at the opposite side. The eggs release a free-swimming miracidium when hatched.

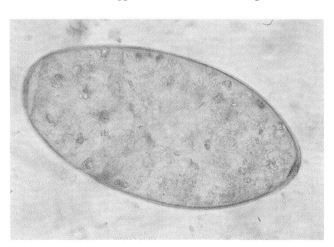

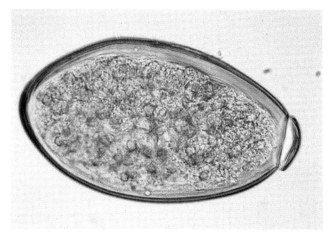

**15-91, 92** *Fasciola hepatica.* **Egg. Feces. Iodine stain (×500).** The unembryonated eggs of *F. hepatica* are large, elongated, and measure 150 × 80 μm. The shell is thin with a small operculum that is difficult to see. The operculum can easily be opened by applying pressure to the coverslip (15-92). The adult worms are large, measuring 30 × 15 mm, and live in the liver and bile duct where they produce eggs that are discharged into the feces.

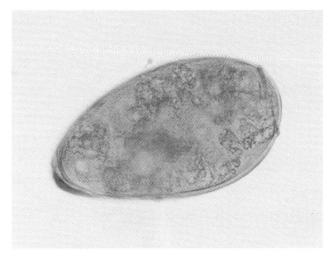

**15-93** *Paragonimus westermani.* **Egg. Feces. Iodine stain (×800).** These eggs are large, usually 100 × 50 μm, oval, with a thick shell and a well-defined operculum at the broad end. The opposite end is thickened but lacks a knob such as the one present in *Diphyllobothrium latum* eggs. The adult fluke lives in the lungs of humans and measures 10 × 5 mm (not shown).

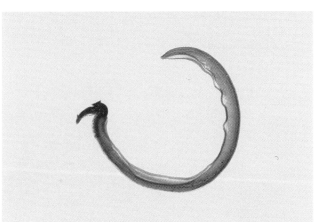

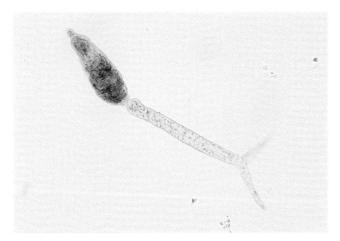

**15-94, 95** *Schistosoma japonicum.* **Carmine stain. Adult male (15-94, ×10) and cercaria (15-95, ×225).** The adult schistosomes reside in blood vessels (Figure 15-94). The eggs produced by the adult female after reaching the water release miracidia that infect specific snails, their intermediate hosts. Following development in the snail, the cercariae (Figure 15-95) emerge and penetrate the skins of humans who are in direct contact with snail-infested water.

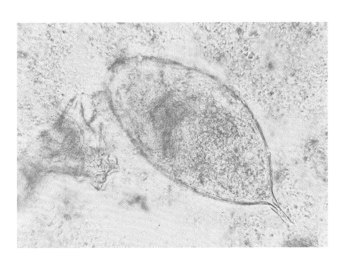

**15-96** *Schistosoma haematobium.* **Egg. Feces. Iodine stain (×600).** These eggs are large, measure 150 × 50 μm, and have a transparent shell with a conspicuous terminal spine.

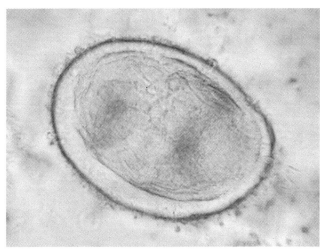

**15-97** *Schistosoma japonicum.* **Egg. Feces. Iodine stain (×700).** The embryonated eggs of *S. japonicum* are ovoid, measure 90 × 50 μm, and have a thin shell and a small spine.

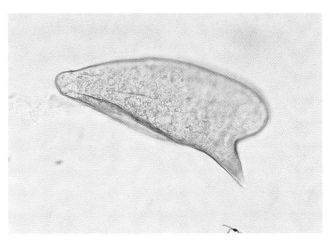 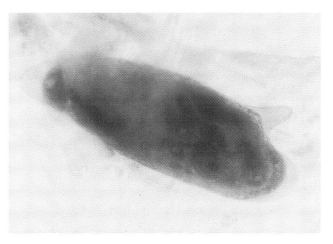

**15-98, 99  *Schistosoma mansoni.* Egg. Feces. Iodine stain (×500).** The eggs of *S. mansoni* are large, 150 × 60 μm, elongated with a thin shell and a distinctive lateral spine. At the time that the eggs are passed in the feces, they contain a miracidium that in fresh preparations can be seen moving. In iodine preparations, the miracidium may stain dark (Figure 15-99).

# Cestodes

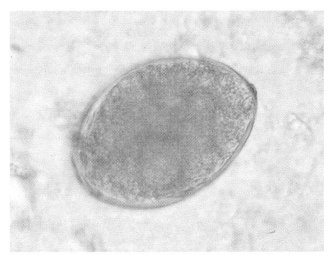 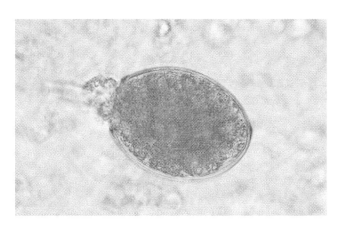

**15-100, 101  *Diphyllobothrium latum.* Egg. Feces. Iodine stain (×800).** The eggs of *D. latum* are ovoid, measure 60 × 50 μm, and have a relatively thick shell. The operculum is not very distinctive, and the small knob located at the opposite end in many instances cannot be observed. The operculum can rupture as shown in Figure 15-101. At the time they are passed in the feces, the eggs are unembryonated. It takes approximately 2 weeks before a ciliated embryo develops.

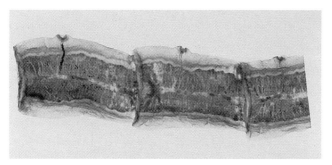

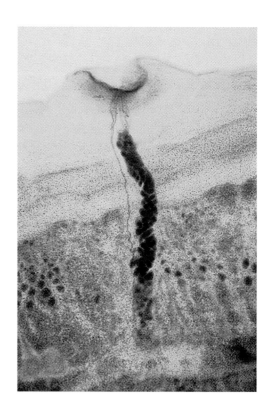

**15-102, 103** *Taenia saginata.* **Proglottids. Carmine stain (15-102, ×5, 15-103, ×16).** The gravid proglottids measure approximately 18 mm in length × 5 to 7 mm in width with the genital pore located at the lateral margin. The proglottids passed in the feces can be identified by injecting India ink through the lateral genital pore and counting the number of primary lateral branches of the uterus. Proglottids with 13 or fewer branches belong to *T. solium*, while those with more than 15 lateral branches are *T. saginata*.

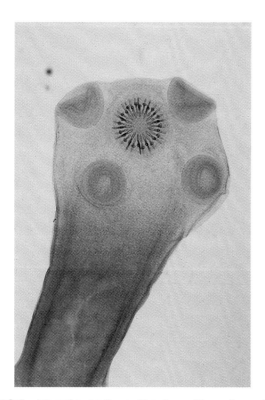

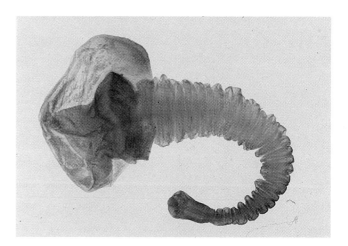

**15-104** *Taenia solium.* **Scolex. Carmine stain (×16).** The scolex of *T. solium* measures 1 mm in diameter, has four suckers, and a rostellum with two rows of hooks. The adult worm can measure up to 5 meters. The life cycle is similar to that of *T. saginata*, although the eggs are directly infectious to humans.

**15-105** *Taenia solium.* **Cysticercus. Carmine stain (×15).** Infections of humans with *T. solium* occur in areas where pigs are bred. Ingestion of the eggs of *T. solium* may result in cysticercosis. The eggs hatch in the small intestine and release oncospheres, which are carried in the bloodstream to distant tissues, where they mature into cysticerci. Cysts containing cysticerci may be formed in the central nervous system, skin, muscle, and skin. These cysts are usually 1 to 4 cm in diameter and are filled with a clear fluid and a single scolex that is invaginated.

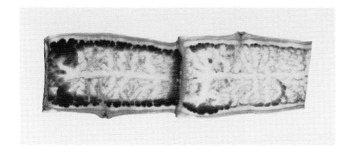

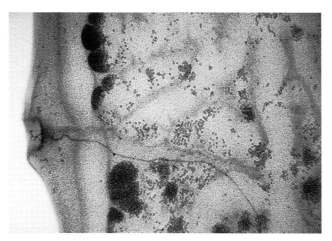

**15-106, 107** *Taenia solium* **proglottids. Carmine stain. (15-106, ×5) (15-107, ×15).**
The gravid proglottids of *T. solium* have fewer than 13 lateral branches on each side of the uterine central core. These proglottids measure around 10 mm in length by 5 mm in width.

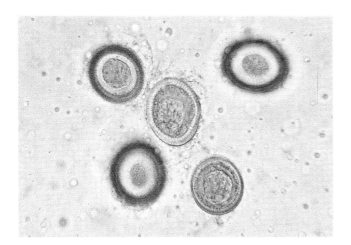

**15-108** *Taenia* **spp. Eggs. Iodine stain (×500).**
The eggs of *T. saginata* and *T. solium* are spherical, measuring approximately 40 μm in diameter. The shell is thick with a radial striation and can stain quite dark. In fresh eggs, a thin outer membrane can occasionally be observed. Inside the egg there is a six-hooked embryo. It is important to be able to observe these six hooks for final identification. These eggs have the same morphology as those of *Echinococcus* spp. The eggs of *T. saginata* are not infectious to humans, in contrast to those of *T. solium*. The eggs of *T. saginata* are ingested by cattle, and after several months they develop in the muscles into cysticerci, which are infectious for humans.

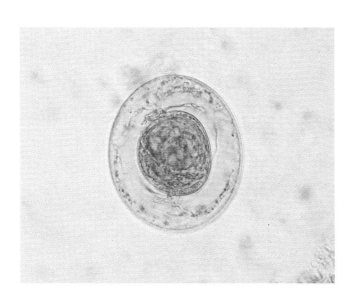

**15-109** *Hymenolepis nana*. **Egg. Feces. Iodine stain (×1000).** The eggs of *H. nana* are spherical to oval and measure 30 to 45 μm in diameter. The shell is thin, and the inner envelope has two polar thickenings that give rise to four to eight filaments located between the embryo and the shell. The embryo, or oncosphere, has six hooks.

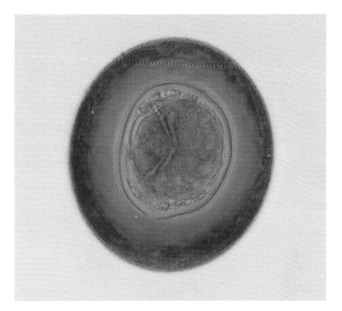

**15-110** *Hymenolepis diminuta.* **Egg. Feces. Iodine (×800).** These eggs are oval, large, measuring 80 × 70 μm, with a thick shell and an inner membrane that surrounds the oncosphere. The oncosphere has six hooks and is surrounded by a membrane that does not have polar filaments.

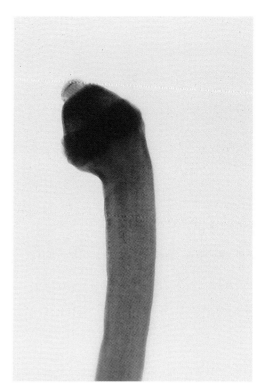

**15-111** *Dipylidium caninum.* **Scolex. Carmine stain (×80).** The scolex of this microorganism contains four large suckers and a conical, retractile rostellum with several rows of small spines.

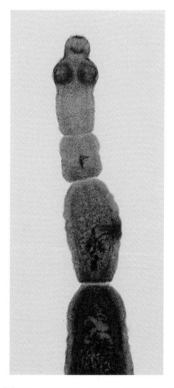

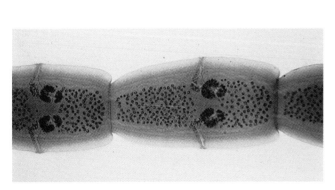

**15-112** *Dipylidium caninum.* **Proglottids. Carmine stain (×15).** Dogs are the usual host of this parasite, but humans can acquire the disease by ingestion of infected fleas. The adult tapeworms measure up to 70 cm. The gravid proglottids measure 25 × 8 mm, and are divided into sections, each containing approximately 10 eggs with six hooks. Typically these proglottids have two genital pores, one on each lateral margin. The eggs can be found occasionally in the feces.

**15-113** *Echinococcus granulosus.* **Adult worm. Carmine stain (×50).** The adult worm of the canine tapeworm *E. granulosus* measures 4 to 6 mm in length, has a scolex with four suckers and a rostellum with hooklets, and three to five proglottids, one of them immature, one mature, and one or two gravid. Dogs release eggs in the feces, which are then ingested by cattle, sheep, and other animals. Humans acquire the disease following accidental ingestion of *E. granulosus* eggs.

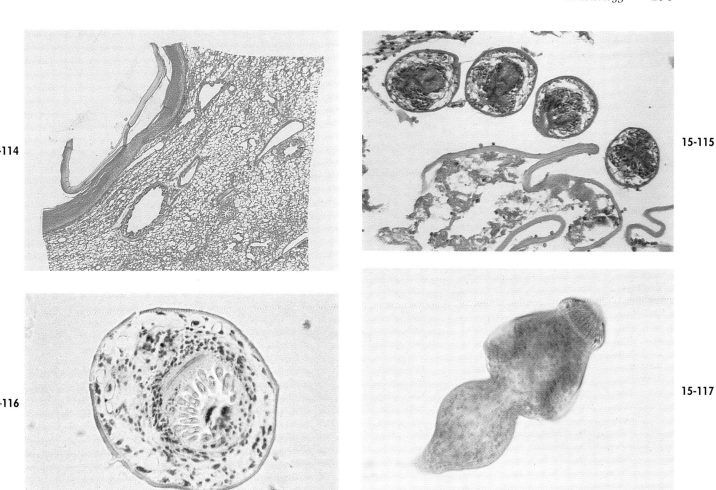

**15-114–117** *Echinococcus granulosus.* **Liver. Hematoxylin and eosin stain (×300).** Hydatid cysts are found in humans mainly in the liver and lung. They consist of an outer wall with a laminated, non-nucleated layer, and an inner layer called *germinative membrane* that is nucleated (Figure 15-114). The germinal layer gives rise to brood capsules with scoleces. Degeneration of these structures results in a fluid material known as hydatid sand (Figure 15-115). In this figure, it is possible to see the wall of the hydatid cyst and four brood capsules with protoscolex. The scoleces are invaginated in their own bodies. At higher magnification, it is possible to observe the rostellum with the hooklets (Figure 15-116). Placing the hydatid sand in saline may cause the scoleces to evaginate (Figure 15-117).

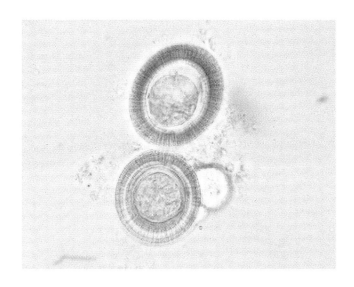

**15-118** *Echinococcus granulosus.* **Eggs. Iodine stain (×800).** The eggs of *E. granulosus* are identical to the eggs of the *Taenia* spp. They are spherical with a thick, radially striated shell and measure 30 to 40 μm in diameter.

# Structures Frequently Found in the Feces that Require Differentiation from Parasites

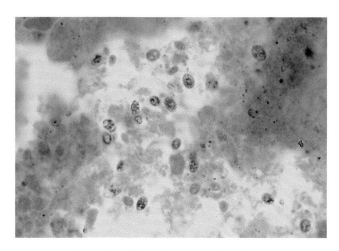 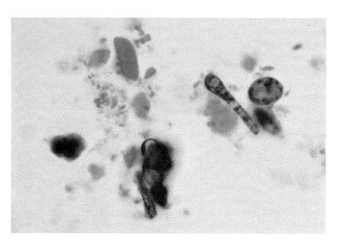

**15-119, 120   Yeast cells. Feces. Trichrome stain (×1250).** Yeast cells are usually round to oval and may stain different colors ranging from green to blue to red, depending on status of the wall of the microorganism.

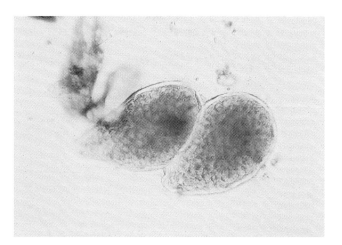 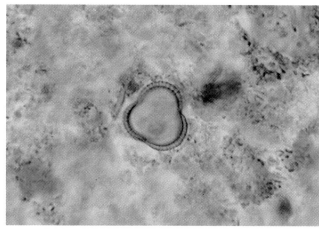

**15-121, 122   Plant cells (15-121: wet mount) and pollen grains (15-122: Trichrome stain). Feces (×1250).** Plant cells and pollen grains can frequently be seen in fecal specimens. The plant cells can widely vary in size and morphology (Figure 15-121). Pollen usually ranges in size from 15 to 60 μm and has a natural brown to green color since it does not pick up the stain. The wall may be smooth or, as in this case, may have a radiated structure (Figure 15-122).

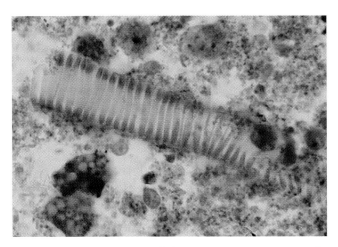

**15-123 Plantar spiral. Feces. Trichrome stain (×1250).** These structures are part of the spirovascular bundle of vegetables and are frequently found in the feces. They can have different sizes and degrees of coiling, and should not be confused with parasites.

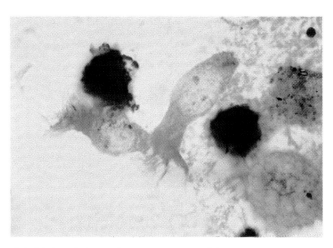

**15-124 Ciliated columnar epithelial cell. Bronchoalveolar lavage. Trichrome stain (×1250).** Epithelial cells from the respiratory mucosa can be seen relatively frequently in pulmonary specimens. The morphology may vary depending on how well the specimen was preserved.

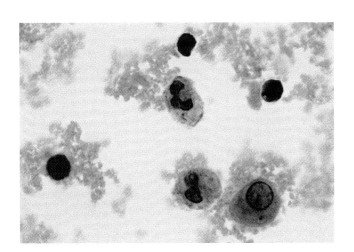

**15-125 White blood cells. Feces. Trichrome stain (×500).** Polymorphonuclear leukocytes and mononuclear cells can be observed in stool specimens. These cells can be confused with members of the *Entamoeba* spp. It is important to consider the size, the ratio of the nucleus to the cytoplasm (usually close to 1:1 in the white cells), and the internal structure of the nucleus. Degenerated macrophages that have ingested debris, including red blood cells, may be particularly difficult to differentiate from *E. histolytica.*

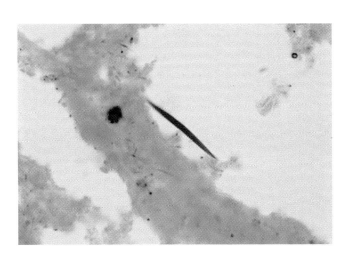

**15-126 Charcot-Leyden crystals. Feces. Trichrome stain (×1250).** These crystals are by-products of eosinophils and are commonly found in patients with parasitic and allergic diseases. With the trichrome stain they usually stain a red color.

# CHAPTER 16 *Virology*

Viruses are the most common cause of human disease. Because of the difficulty in growing them in culture, they have only recently begun to be understood. In contrast to other microbes, mature viruses contain only one type of nucleic acid. DNA viruses that infect humans include pox viruses, some hepatitis viruses, wart viruses, and herpes viruses. RNA viruses include poliovirus, rabies virus, influenza virus, mumps virus, and many others. Viruses also have a protein coat, called a capsid, and some viruses may acquire a lipid envelope during migration from an infected cell or from the nucleus to the cytoplasm of a cell.

Viruses are either detected directly in clinical material using antigen detection tests including immunoserological stains and nucleic acid detection methods, or they are cultured in cells and recognized by their damage to the cells, called cytopathic effect (CPE). Antibodies to infecting viruses are also often used to diagnose viral infections.

## Instrumentation and Equipment

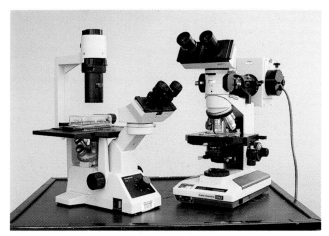

**16-1 Microscopes (Olympus Optical Co., Ltd., Japan).** A brightfield microscope equipped with epiluminescence is shown on the right and an inverted microscope is on the left. The fluorescence microscope is frequently used in the virology laboratory for the examination of clinical specimens and viruses in culture using immunofluorescent stains. The inverted microscope illuminates the sample from the top, with the objectives underneath the specimen. This configuration allows the examination of the cell monolayer from the bottom of the container, while the cells are covered by the nutrient medium. Inverted microscopes are particularly useful for the examination of tissue culture cells in bottles, flasks, microtiter plates, and tubes.

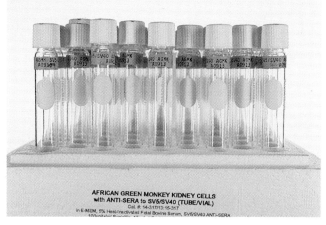

**16-2 Rack with tissue culture tubes.** Different types of cell monolayers already seeded in tubes can be purchased from commercial companies, or can be prepared in the laboratory. The monolayers grow on the side of the tube that is covered with tissue culture medium when the tube is on its side during incubation. The rack is placed inside a 33° to 37°C incubator after clinical specimens have been inoculated into the tube. The monolayers are observed under an inverted microscope for the presence of CPE.

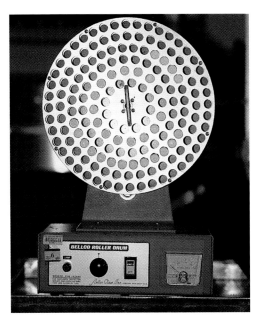

**16-3 Roller drum (Bellco Glass, Inc., Vineland, N.J.).** This instrument holds, and continuously rotates, tubes containing cell lines. The drum is placed inside an incubator at 33°–37°C. The holder containing the tubes can be removed from the incubator so that the tubes can be checked for CPE. This apparatus is most frequently used for culturing respiratory specimens for viruses such as influenza and parainfluenza.

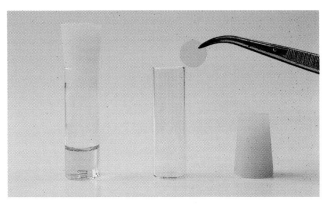

**16-4 Shell vial.** A shell vial is a $15 \times 45$ mm glass vial containing culture medium and a round 12 to 13 mm glass coverslip on which a monolayer of cells has been cultivated. To inoculate a clinical specimen, the medium is discarded, the specimen is added to the vial on top of the monolayer, and the vial is centrifuged. At the completion of the centrifugation, fresh culture medium is added and the vial is capped and incubated. Specimens suspected of containing certain viruses, including cytomegalovirus, herpes simplex virus, varicella zoster virus, and the bacterium *Chlamydia* spp., among others, are processed using this technique since it shortens the time for identification of the pathogen and may increase the recovery.

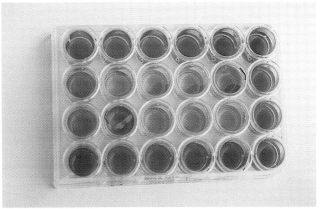

**16-5 Multiple well plates.** Plastic plates with 24, 48, or 96 wells are used instead of shell vials by some laboratories for the isolation of viruses and *Chlamydia* from clinical specimens. The main advantage of these plates is that they allow for the simultaneous processing of multiple specimens. Problems include the possibility of cross-contamination between specimens and a lower sensitivity of the assay due to, at least in part, the decrease in sample volume.

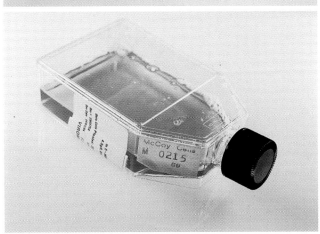

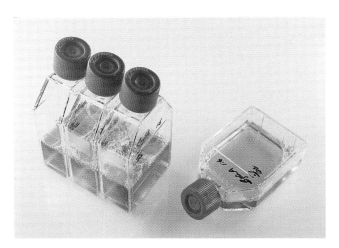

**16-6, 7 Tissue culture flasks.** Plastic or glass flasks of different sizes can be utilized to grow cell monolayers or cells in suspension. Once the flasks are seeded, they are placed inside incubators.

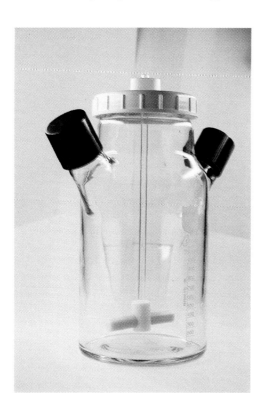

**16-8  Spinner bottles.** This type of bottle is used for producing large quantities of viruses in cells that are grown in suspension. In the center of the bottle there is a magnetic stir bar. When the bottle is placed on a stirring apparatus, the magnetic bar spins around and maintains the cells in suspension. The CPE can be visualized by taking an aliquot of the suspended cells and observing them under the microscope.

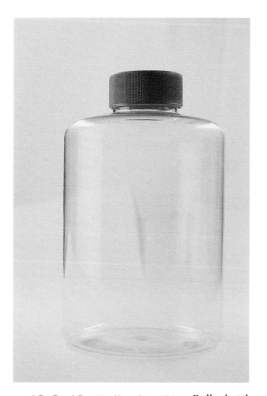

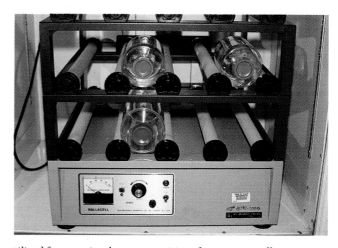

**16-9, 10  Roller bottles.** Roller bottles are also utilized for growing large quantities of viruses in cell monolayers (Figure 16-9). The cells are seeded into the bottle with medium and the bottles are placed in a roller bottle apparatus (Figure 16-10) located inside an incubator that continuously rotates the bottles. Once the cells are attached in a monolayer around the interior walls of the bottle, the viral inoculum is added and the bottle placed back on the rotating module (New Brunswick Scientific, Edison, N. J.). The cells can be harvested when the desired CPE is observed in the cell monolayer.

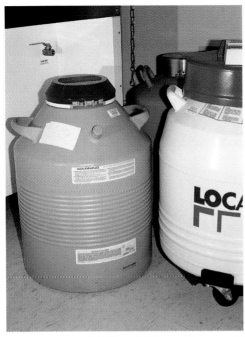

**16-11 Liquid nitrogen tanks (Union Carbide Cryogenic Equipment, Danbury, Ct.).** Liquid nitrogen containers are used for the long-term preservation of tissue culture cells and viruses. Specimens and isolates stored under liquid nitrogen, with a temperature of $-195°C$, can be maintained in a viable state for indefinite periods of time. Although liquid nitrogen tanks are self-contained, (i.e., they do not need electricity to maintain the temperature) they need to be replenished with liquid nitrogen on a regular basis because the nitrogen is continuously being lost due to evaporation.

## Detection and Identification of Viruses

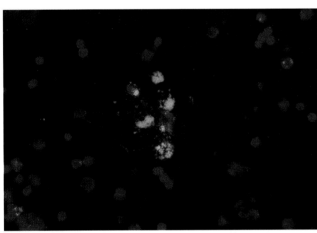

**16-12 Adenoviridae. Adenovirus. Direct fluorescent assay. Nasopharyngeal swab (×300).** For the direct detection of adenovirus-infected cells, a mouse monoclonal anti-adenovirus antibody is layered onto and incubated with the fresh specimen on a slide. A goat antimouse fluorescein-labeled conjugate with Evans blue counterstain is then added. As shown here, positive specimens have an apple-green stippled staining of the nucleus.

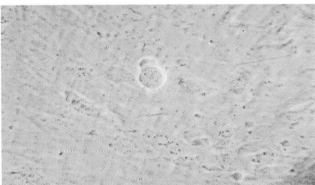
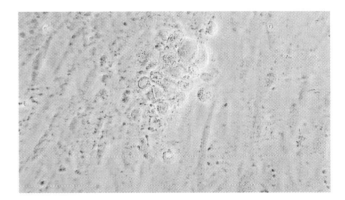

**16-13, 14 Adenoviridae. Adenovirus. MRC-5 cells. Cytopathic effect (CPE). Phase contrast (×225).** Adenoviruses grow well in a variety of human cell lines such as HeLa, HEp-2, KB, A549, and can also be isolated in primary human kidney cells and in fetal diploid fibroblast, such as MRC-5, cell cultures. Typically the initial CPE appears at 3 to 5 days and consists of rounding of individual cells (Figure 16-13) that subsequently become significantly enlarged and refractile, giving the appearance of balloons. As the CPE continues and involves the surrounding cells, it forms grapelike clusters (Figure 16-14). The CPE usually spreads to the rest of the monolayer over a period of days.

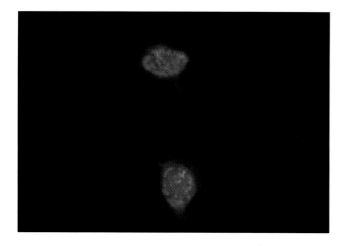

**16-15   Adenoviridae. Adenovirus. MRC-5 cells. Culture identification. Fluorescent stain (×500).** To confirm the identification of an adenovirus, fluorescein-labeled monoclonal antibodies can be used. Here fluorescence is visible both in the cytoplasm and the nucleus of the infected cells. Adenoviruses replicate in the nucleus where bright fluorescent dots can be observed.

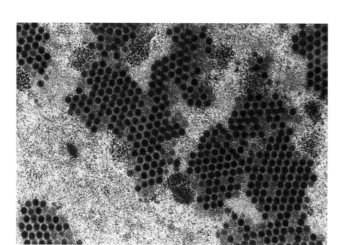

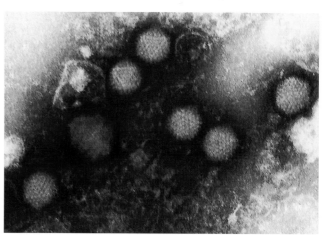

**16-16, 17   Adenoviridae. Adenovirus. Electron microscopy. Transmission (16-16, ×27,500) and negative staining (16-17, ×100,000).** Tissues or cells suspected of containing adenoviruses can be fixed, cut, and stained for observation by transmission electron microscopy. Adenoviruses can form crystalline arrays in the nucleus of the cell (Figure 16-16). Urine and feces specimens can be clarified and observed using the negative-staining technique, in which the background is stained dark to reveal the unstained virus particles (Figure 16-17). Adenoviruses measure 60 to 90 nm in diameter, do not have an envelope, are of cubic symmetry, and possess a capsid composed of 252 capsomers, each approximately 7 to 9 nm in diameter.

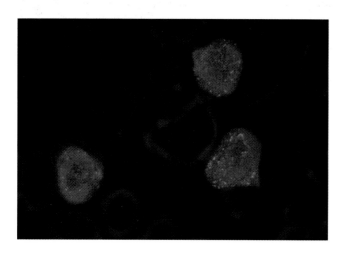

**16-18   Adenoviridae. Adenovirus. Antibody detection. Fluorescent assay (×800).** Several techniques can be used for the detection of antibodies to adenoviruses including complement fixation tests, hemagglutination inhibition, enzyme immunoassays, and fluorescent methods. This figure shows the detection of antibodies to adenoviruses using an indirect immunofluorescent assay. Human epithelial cells are infected with adenovirus, mixed with non-infected cells, and then the cells are fixed to a glass slide. The serum from the patient is incubated with the specimen and washed; an antihuman fluorescein-labeled globulin is then added, and the specimen is observed using a fluorescence microscope. If antibody is present, as in this case, infected cells fluoresce apple-green.

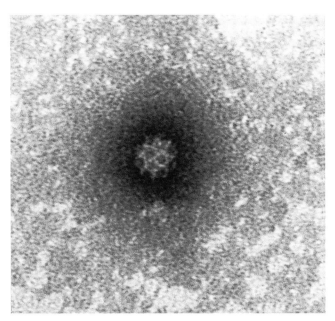

**16-19 Caliciviridae. Calicivirus. Feces. Electron microscopy. Negative staining (×400,000).** Caliciviruses have been identified as a frequent cause of gastroenteritis in young children. Diagnosis requires electron microscopy or immunoserological testing. These virions are spherical, 35 to 40 nm in diameter, with 32 cup-shaped depressions and icosahedral symmetry.

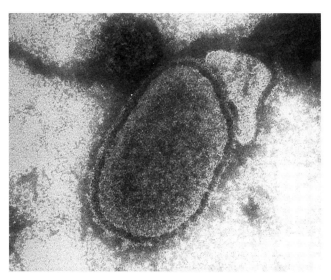

**16-20 Coronaviridae. Coronavirus. Feces. Electron microscopy. Negative staining (×100,000).** Coronaviruses have been associated with acute upper respiratory tract infections in children and diarrheal illnesses in children and adults. Identification of these viruses requires electron microscopy studies or culture in human embryonic trachea tissue cultures. The coronaviruses are enveloped, pleomorphic particles that measure 80 to 120 nm in diameter. This family of viruses is named for the club-shaped peplomers (virally encoded proteins) that project from the envelope and that, as shown here, form a thin border resembling a "solar corona" under electron microscopic examination of negatively stained preparations.

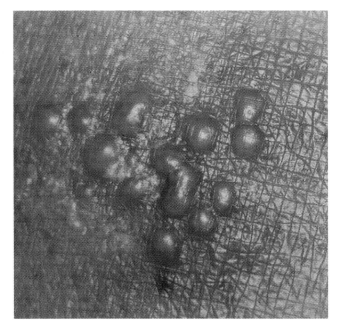

**16-21 Herpesviridae. Herpes simplex virus (HSV). Skin lesions.** HSV-1, in general, produces infections in the upper part of the body, while HSV-2 is frequently isolated from sites below the waist, including the genital area. Skin and mucocutaneous lesions, in the form of fluid-filled vesicles approximately 2 to 5 mm in diameter, evolve over a period of 7 to 14 days. At the time that vesicles are present, direct antigen detection from scrapings of tissue at the vesicle base using monoclonal antibodies is a highly specific and sensitive method.

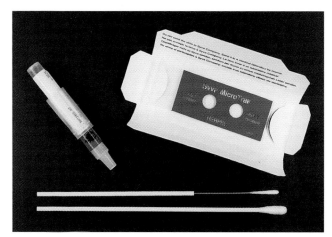

**16-22 Herpesviridae. Herpes simplex virus (HSV). Direct antigen test kit (Syva, Co., San Jose, Calif.).** A system frequently used for the detection of certain pathogens, such as HSV and *Chlamydia trachomatis*, is shown in this slide. Swabs are provided for collecting specimens from the eye, the female cervix and the male urethra, or other body sites. Once the specimen is collected, the swab is rolled onto the glass slide and fixative is added. The slide, enclosed in the provided container, is then submitted to the laboratory for staining with a fluorescein-labeled monoclonal antibody.

**16-23 Herpesviridae. Herpes simplex virus (HSV). Direct immunofluorescent assay (DFA) (×500).** Direct staining with a specific monoclonal antibody of infected cells collected from the base of HSV vesicle allows for the rapid detection and identification of this virus. Although this technique may be overall less sensitive than culture, it has the advantage that a viable virus is not required for obtaining a positive result. An additional advantage is that the test results are available shortly after collecting the specimen. As shown in this DFA-stained slide, infected cells show an apple-green fluorescence in both cytoplasm and nucleus.

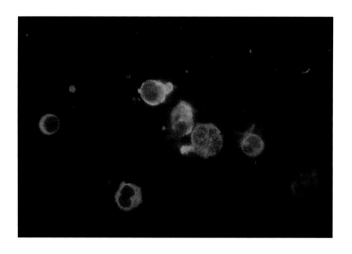

**16-24 Herpesviridae. Herpes simplex virus. Cervical swab. Horseradish peroxidase stain (×300).** Cervical specimens, collected as for Pap smears, can be stained with specific antibodies to HSV. As shown here, infected cells stained with horseradish peroxidase have a brown color.

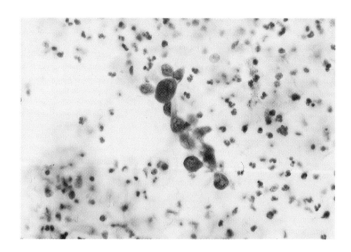

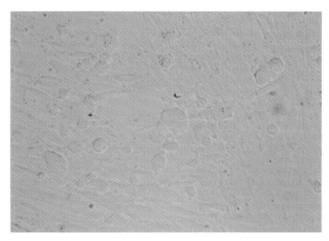 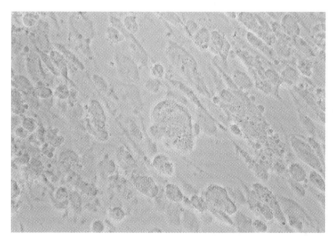

**16-25, 26 Herpesviridae. Herpes simplex virus (HSV). MRC-5 cells. CPE seen under phase contrast (×225).** HSV 1 and 2 grow rapidly *in vitro*, producing CPE in 24 to 48 hours. Several cell lines can be used to isolate and identify these viruses, including human diploid fibroblasts such as MRC-5 or WI-38, and primary rabbit kidney cells. As shown in Figure 16-25, early CPE is characterized by large, round cells appearing as localized foci in several areas of the monolayer. The CPE progresses rapidly and by 3 to 5 days usually involves the entire monolayer. Occasionally, formation of multinucleated syncytial giant cells can be observed (Figure 16-26).

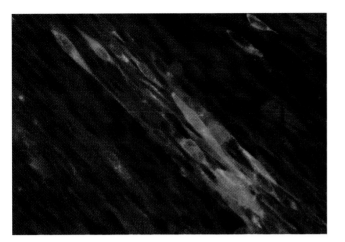
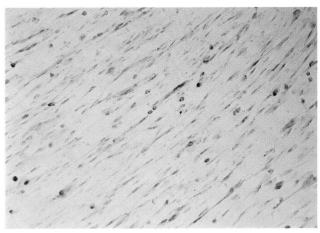

**16-27, 28  Herpesviridae. Herpes simplex virus (HSV). MRC-5 cells. Shell vial culture. Fluorescein (16-27, ×300) and horseradish peroxidase stains (16-28, ×225).** The monolayers were stained after 48 hours of incubation. After fixation, a fluorescein-labeled monoclonal antibody (Figure 16-27) or a horseradish peroxidase-labeled antibody (Figure 16-28) was used to detect the infected cells. Specific monoclonal antibodies to HSV 1 and 2 can be used separately or in combination, thus allowing for typing of the isolate.

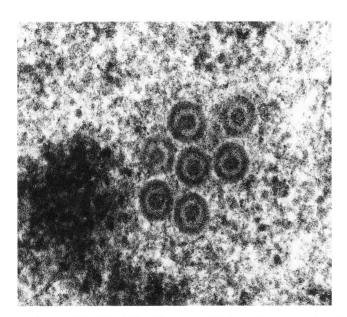
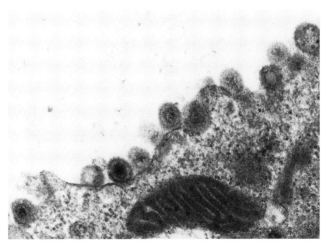

**16-29, 30  Herpesviridae. Herpes simplex virus (HSV). Transmission electron microscopy (16-29, ×100,000; 16-30, ×35,500).** The family of Herpesviridae has several members that are frequent human pathogens, including HSV 1 and 2, cytomegalovirus, varicella zoster virus, and Epstein Barr virus, in addition to the recently discovered HSV 6, HSV 7, and HSV 8. All have a similar morphological structure consisting of a cylindrical core containing the viral DNA, an icosahedral capsid that measures 90 to 110 nm in diameter, a granular zone that surrounds the capsid, and an external envelope. The complete viral particle measures 180 to 200 nm in diameter. As shown in Figure 16-29, the viral particles form in the host cell nucleus, but the envelope is acquired at the time of budding through the cellular membrane (Figure 16-30).

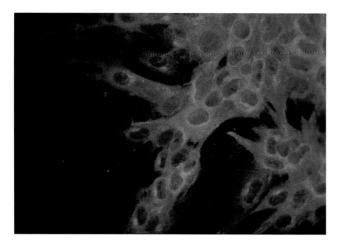

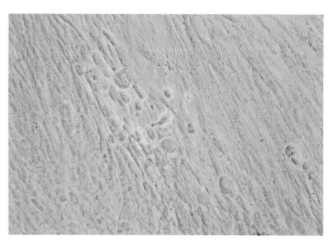

**16-31 Herpesviridae. Herpes simplex virus (HSV). Antibody detection. Fluorescent stain (×225).** Human diploid cells infected with HSV 1 or 2 can be used as substrate to detect antibodies to these viruses in human serum. There is a significant amount of cross reactivity between antibodies to HSV 1 and HSV 2 and thus, these tests should not be used to identify the specific virus causing the infection. Western blot analysis and detection of antibodies to specific HSV 1 and HSV 2 antigens are now available for that purpose.

**16-32 Herpesviridae. Cytomegalovirus (CMV). MRC-5 cells. CPE seen under phase contrast (×225).** CMV has species-specific growth requirements; thus, human diploid fibroblast cells, either MRC-5 or WI-38, are used for culture. The foci of CPE are slow to appear but usually are visible by 5 to 10 days, so cultures should be maintained for up to 21 days. CPE is characterized by the presence of round, large, refractile cells in elongated foci parallel to the long axis of the monolayer. The CPE spreads slowly and, as a result, the surrounding cells maintain a normal morphology for extended periods of time. In most instances, unless the initial inoculum is large, the entire monolayer is not involved.

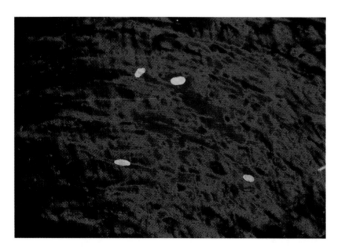

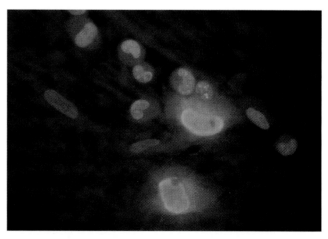

**16-33, 34 Herpesviridae. Cytomegalovirus (CMV). MRC-5 cells. Shell vial. Immunofluorescent stain (×500).** The use of the shell vial centrifugation method has allowed early detection of CMV in clinical specimens. Following centrifugation of the specimen onto the monolayer, the culture is incubated for 24 to 48 hours at 37°C and subsequently stained with a monoclonal antibody to one of the early CMV antigens. As shown in Figure 16-33, staining of the nuclei occurs early, before cytopathic effect can be detected. Monolayers stained at a later time after infection show both nuclear and cytoplasmic fluorescence. Early CPE can be observed in Figure 16-34.

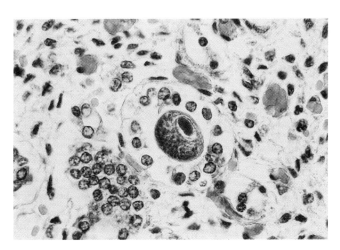
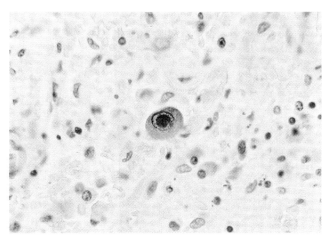

**16-35, 36  Herpesviridae. Cytomegalovirus (CMV). 16-35; Kidney. Hematoxylin and eosin (H&E) stain (×500). 16-36; Lung. Horseradish peroxidase (HRP) stain (×500).** Tissues infected with CMV may have nuclear and cytoplasmic inclusions. The most characteristic nuclear inclusions have the appearance of an "owl's eye" as a result of the retraction of the tissue, producing the clear halo. Granular eosinophilic inclusions in the cytoplasm are not so distinctive. These inclusions are visible in H&E stained preparations (Figure 16-35) but the use of specific antibodies labeled with HRP allow for a more specific and sensitive identification (Figure 16-36).

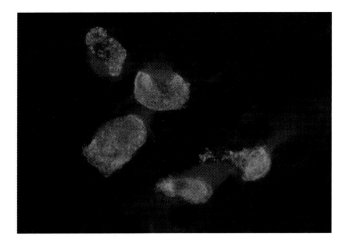

**16-37  Herpesviridae. Cytomegalovirus (CMV). Antibody detection. Immunofluorescent assay (×500).** Monolayers of human fibroblasts are infected with CMV for use as the substrate for this assay. It is important to have a mixture of infected and noninfected cells in the monolayer in order to be able to discriminate between specific and nonspecific staining. The specific CMV staining should be mainly nuclear, as shown here. Seroconversion from a negative to a positive status is a good indication of a primary infection. However, changes in antibody titers should only be interpreted in conjunction with other clinical and laboratory parameters.

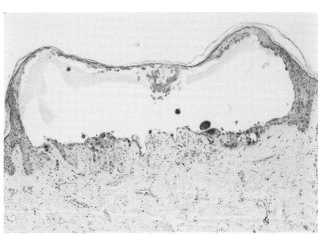
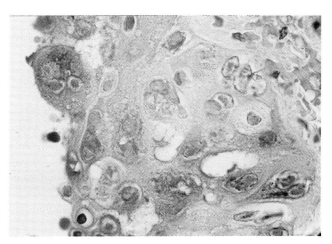

**16-38, 39  Herpesviridae. Varicella zoster virus (VZV). Skin lesions. H&E stain 16-38, ×30 and 16-39, ×500.** Intraepidermal vesicle resulting from a VZV infection (Figure 16-38). Several multinucleated giant cells with eosinophilic Cowdry type A (typical intranuclear) inclusions are visible (Figure 16-39).

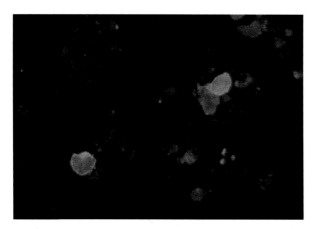

**16-40  Herpesviridae.  Varicella zoster virus (VZV).  Skin  lesion.  Direct  fluorescent  assay (×300).** Specific monoclonal antibodies can be used for the identification of VZV infected cells in clinical samples. As shown here, fluorescein-tagged antibodies produce apple-green fluorescence in the nucleus and cytoplasm of the infected cells.

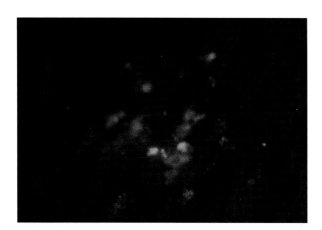

**16-42  Herpesviridae.  Varicella  zoster  virus (VZV).  Shell  vial.  Fluorescent  stain  (×500).** Human diploid lung cells are used to prepare shell vials for the detection of VZV. Commercially available fluorescein-conjugated monoclonal antibodies are used to stain the monolayer 48 to 72 hours after inoculation. This method greatly facilitates the identification of VZV and speeds up the process by several days compared with waiting for CPE. Nuclear and cytoplasmic fluorescence can be observed in this slide.

**16-44  Herpesviridae.  Epstein-Barr  virus (EBV).  Commercial  particle  agglutination  test for serological diagnosis.** EBV does not readily grow in tissue culture; therefore, the diagnosis of an EBV infection is frequently made using serological tests. A screening test for heterophile antibodies, IgM antibodies that react with antigens that are not related to the organism producing the antibody response, is positive in most patients with infectious mononucleosis. A latex agglutination test, "Monospot-type" test (Figure 16-44, Biokit USA, Inc., Lexington, Mass.), is often used to detect heterophile antibodies.

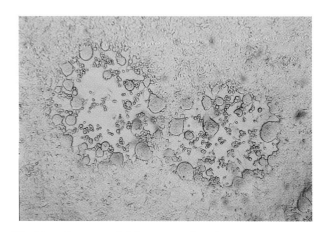

**16-41  Herpesviridae.  Varicella  zoster  virus (VZV).  A549  cells.  CPE  seen  under  phase  contrast (×225).** Human diploid fibroblast cell cultures are used in most laboratories for the isolation and identification of VZV. The CPE produced is slow to appear and does not spread readily to the rest of the monolayer. The cultures should be maintained for 21 days before they are discarded. Figure 16-41 shows VZV CPE in A549 cells, in which the initial CPE consists of swollen, refractile cells. As the CPE progresses, it acquires a doughnutlike shape containing a center of necrotic cells surrounded by large, refractile, giant cells. Spread of the foci occurs by infection of adjacent cells, since the virus is highly cell-associated.

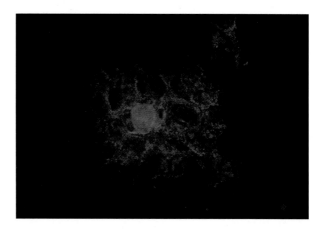

**16-43  Herpesviridae.  Varicella  zoster  virus. Antibody  detection.  Immunofluorescent  assay (×300).** Cells infected with VZV can be used as the antigen in an indirect immunofluorescent test for the presence of antibodies to this virus.

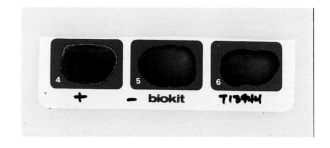

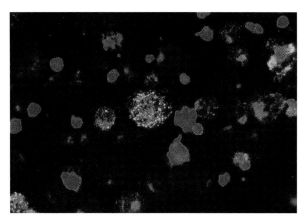
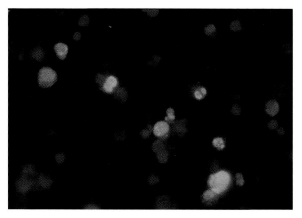

**16-45, 46 Immunofluorescent tests for antibodies to Epstein-Barr virus structural antigens.** Detection of antibodies to specific antigens of EBV can be accomplished using cell lines infected with EBV as substrates for indirect immunofluorescent methods. P3HR-1 cells expressing the EBV viral capsid antigen (VCA) are used for detecting IgM (Figure 16-45) and IgG (Figure 16-46) antibodies to VCA.

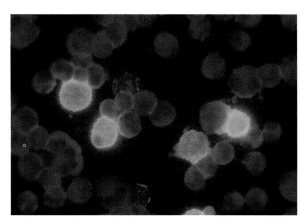
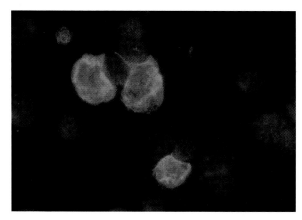

**16-47, 48 Immunofluorescent tests for antibodies to Epstein-Barr virus early antigens.** Antibodies to two types of early antigens (EA) are seen in infected Raji cells: diffuse (D), in which the antigen is distributed in the nucleus and cytoplasm (Figure 16-47); and restricted (R), in which the antigen is only in the cytoplasm. Figure 16-48 shows antibodies against both D and R early antigens.

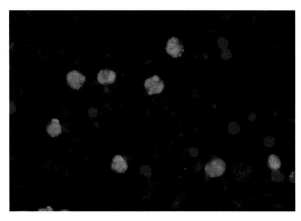
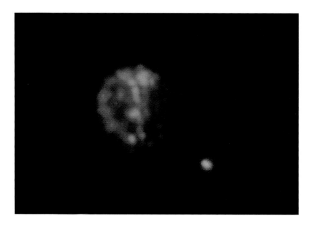

**16-49 Immunofluorescent test for antibodies against nuclear antigen of Epstein-Barr virus (EBNA).** The Raji cell line is also used for the detection of antibodies to EBNA using an anti-complement indirect immunofluorescent staining technique.

**16-50 Orthomyxoviridae. Influenza A. Direct fluorescent assay (×1350).** Nasopharyngeal specimens can be directly stained using fluorescein-labeled monoclonal antibodies to influenza A, B, and C viruses. An apple-green fluorescent granular pattern can be observed in the nucleus of this infected cell.

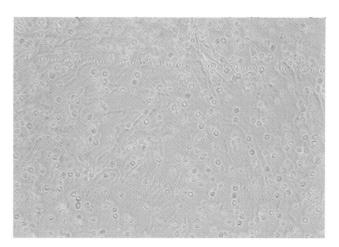 

**16-51, 52  Orthomyxoviridae. Influenza A. African green monkey kidney cells. Hemadsorption. Phase contrast (×225).** Although in the past, embryonated hens' eggs were used for the isolation of influenza viruses, continuous cells lines are currently utilized in most laboratories. Certain viruses, including influenza, parainfluenza, and mumps viruses, produce glycoproteins that are incorporated into the host cell membrane. Although these viruses cause minimal or no cytopathic effect, guinea pig red blood cells adhere to the host cell membranes when they are added to tissue culture cells infected with these viruses. This phenomenon, termed *hemadsorption*, is demonstrated in Figure 16-51. Figure 16-52 shows a control uninfected monolayer of African green monkey kidney cells.

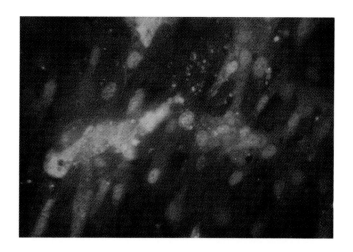

**16-53  Orthomyxoviridae. Influenza. Shell vial. Fluorescent stain (×300).** Inoculation of the specimen into a shell vial followed by staining at 48 to 72 hours with a specific fluorescein-labeled monoclonal antibody allows for the rapid detection and identification of influenza viruses from clinical specimens. Fluorescent staining appears both in the nucleus and cytoplasm of the infected cells.

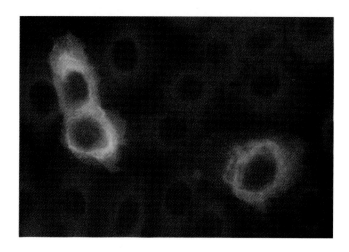

**16-54  Orthomyxoviridae. Influenza. Antibody detection. Immunofluorescent assay, (×500).** Complement fixation, enzyme immunoassays, hemagglutination inhibition, and fluorescent methods are used for the detection of antibodies to influenza viruses. In this slide, a monolayer of cells infected with influenza has been used as a substrate to test for the presence of anti-influenza antibodies using an indirect immunofluorescent method.

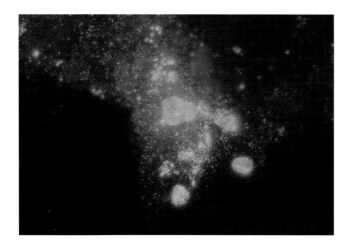

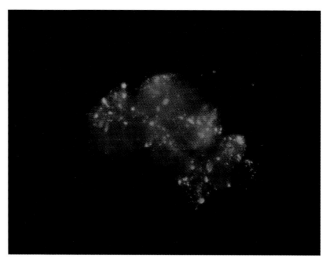

**16-55, 56 Orthomyxoviridae. Parainfluenza 3 (16-55) and 4 (16-56). Nasal washings. Immunofluorescent staining (×500).** Fluorescein-labeled monoclonal antibodies are used for direct staining of clinical specimens for the detection of parainfluenza types 1, 2, 3, and 4 viruses. The fluorescent staining appears predominantly in the cytoplasm of the cells.

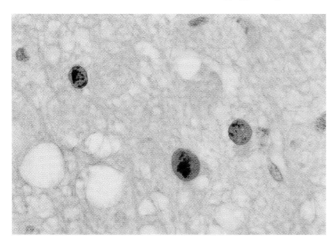

**16-57 Papovaviridae. JC virus. Progressive multifocal leukoencephalopathy (PML). Brain tissue section. Immunoperoxidase stain (×500).** Fluorescent and enzymatic immunostaining methods and nucleic acid probes can be used for the detection of the JC virus in biopsies from patients suspected of having PML. In this case, the infected glial cells stain dark brown.

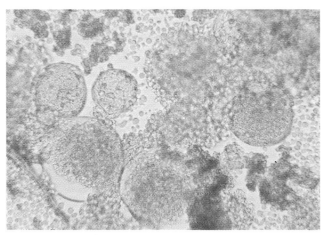

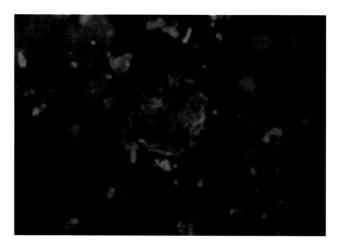

**16-58, 59 Paramyxoviridae. Measles. Phytohemagglutinin stimulated cord blood mononuclear cell culture. CPE; 16-58 (×500). Fluorescent staining; 16-59 (×200).** Primary monkey kidney and Vero cells are frequently used for the isolation of the measles virus. The resulting CPE may consist of spindle-shaped single cells or syncytial multinucleated giant cells. Peripheral blood mononuclear cells have also been used for detection of the measles virus where, as shown in Figure 16-58, formation of giant cells can be observed. The virus responsible for the CPE can be confirmed by staining the culture with fluorescein-labeled antibodies (Figure 16-59).

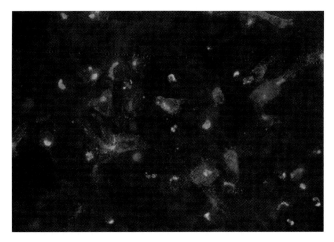

**16-60 Paramyxoviridae. Measles. Vero cell culture. Fluorescent staining (×300).** The measles virus-infected cells are stained with a fluorescent-labeled specific antibody.

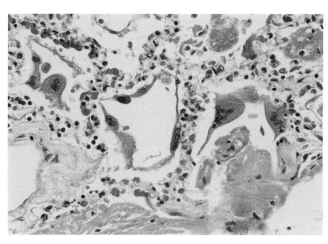

**16-61 Paramyxoviridae. Measles. Lung tissue section. H&E (×500).** Measles virus infections in the lungs can produce a severe pneumonia. The histological section shown here depicts the formation of multinucleated giant cells (Warthin-Finkeldey cells).

**16-62 Paramyxoviridae. Measles. Antibody detection. Indirect immunofluorescent assay (×500).** Antibodies to the measles virus can be detected using different techniques, including complement fixation, indirect fluorescent antibody stains, hemagglutinin inhibition, and enzyme immunoassays. In this slide, a measles-infected cell culture has been incubated with patient serum and stained with a fluorescein-conjugated antihuman immunoglobulin. Either IgG or IgM can be detected in this way.

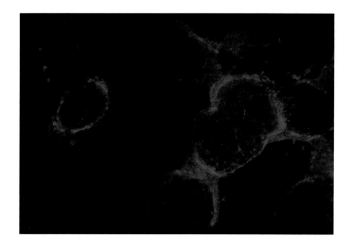

**16-63 Paramyxoviridae. Respiratory syncytial virus (RSV). Direct fluorescent assay (×500).** Fluorescein-labeled monoclonal antibodies can be used for the direct detection of RSV in clinical specimens. Typically an apple-green stippled fluorescence can be observed in the nucleus and cytoplasm of the infected cells, as shown in this slide. RSV is sensitive to temperature and dry conditions and as a result, it quickly loses its viability unless it is collected and transported to the laboratory under optimal conditions. Thus, in certain clinical situations, the direct assays may be more sensitive than culture.

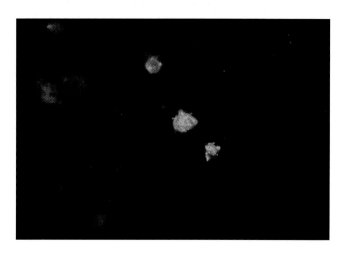

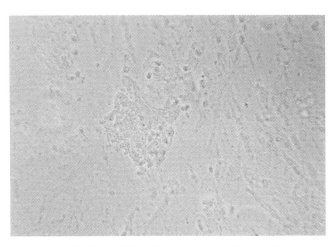
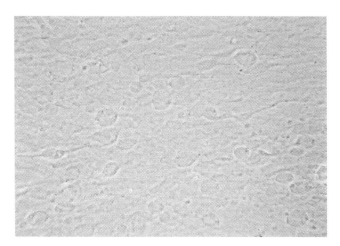

**16-64, 65  Paramyxoviridae. Respiratory syncytial virus. CPE in MRC-5 cells. Phase contrast (×225).** HEp-2, HeLa, and MRC-5 cell lines are frequently used for the isolation of RSV. CPE usually appears by 5 to 10 days and is characterized by the formation of multinucleated giant syncytial cells (Figure 16-64). Occasionally, on heavily positive specimens, CPE may appear by 2 to 4 days; in this case the monolayer may show only rounded up cells that can be confused with a toxic or degenerative effect (Figure 16-65).

**16-66  Paramyxoviridae. Respiratory syncytial virus. MRC-5 cells in shell vial. Culture identification. Fluorescent stain (×300).** RSV can be identified in cell culture using fluorescent-labeled monoclonal antibodies. As shown in this slide, an apple-green bright speckled stain can be observed in the cytoplasm of the infected cells.

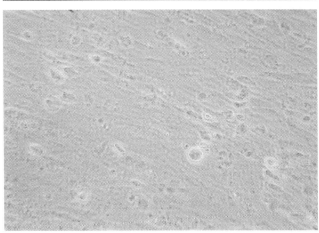
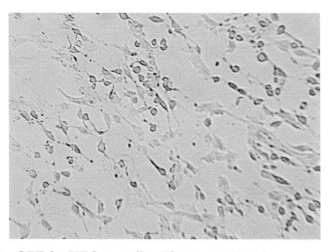

**16-67, 68  Picornaviridae. Echovirus 11. CPE in MRC-5 cells. Phase contrast (×225).** The family Picornaviridae includes four genera: enterovirus, rhinovirus, cardiovirus, and aphthovirus. The first two genera are significant human pathogens. The enteroviruses comprise the coxsackieviruses, echoviruses, and polioviruses. Most of the enteroviruses replicate well in primary monkey kidney cells and produce CPE in 2 to 5 days. As shown in Figure 16-67, the infected cells round up, shrink, and become refractile. The cells quickly degenerate, with marked pyknosis (shrinking) of the nuclei, and detach from the surface of the container (Figure 16-68). Identification of the specific enterovirus isolate is performed by blocking the infectivity with pools of neutralizing sera.

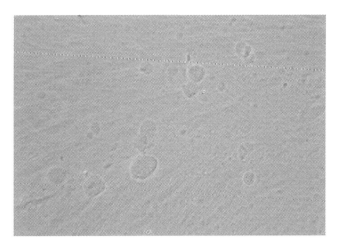

**16-69 Picornaviridae. Rhinovirus. CPE in MRC-5 cells. Phase contrast (×225).** Human diploid fibroblasts are often utilized for the isolation of rhinoviruses from clinical specimens. It is recommended that these cultures be incubated in roller drums inside incubators at 33 to 34°C. The CPE is characterized by the formation of rounded cells of uneven size and a refractile or ground glass appearance. These foci of CPE usually become evident during the first week and subsequently spread throughout the rest of the monolayer.

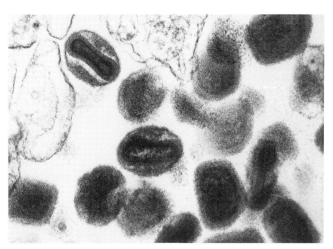

**16-70 Poxviridae. Vaccinia virus. Tissue culture preparation. Transmission electron microscopy (×60,000).** Poxviruses are large and very complex viruses with a typical brick-shape morphology measuring 250 × 200 nm. The internal biconcave core contains the DNA genome. Two lateral bodies are arranged along the concavities of the core, and the virion is surrounded by a viral membrane. Inside the host cell, the virion may have a double membrane that is lost when the virus is extruded from the cell.

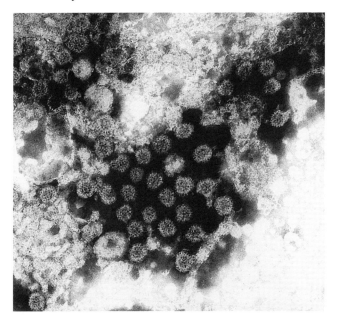

**16-71 Reoviridae. Rotavirus. Feces. Electron microscopy. Negative staining (×100,000).** Rotaviruses are one of the most common agents causing acute gastroenteritis in children. Visualization by electron microscopy was the standard method for detecting these viruses in fecal specimens until sensitive enzyme immunoassays were developed; now EIA is the most frequently used method for diagnosis. Rotavirus particles measure approximately 70 nm in diameter and have the appearance of a wheel, thus the name *Rota* from the Latin word for *wheel*. The core contains 11 segments of double-stranded RNA and is surrounded by a capsid that has 92 capsomers.

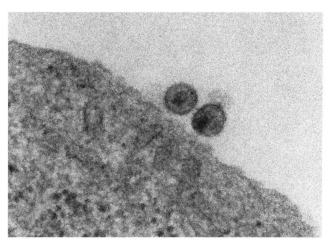

**16-72 Retroviridae. Human immunodeficiency virus type 1 (HIV-1). Tissue culture. Transmission electron microscopy (×100,000).** HIV has a cylindrical core surrounded by the viral envelope. In this slide, transverse sections of the core appear round and electron dense. The virions measure 80 to 100 nm in diameter and have glycoprotein projections, as shown here, that measure 8 to 10 nm in diameter. The virions bud from the cytoplasmic membrane of the host cell. (Special thanks to Dr. Edward Robinson for growing this preparation of HIV-1).

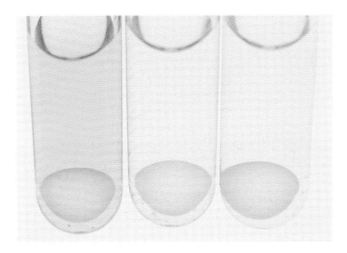

**16-73 Retroviridae. HIV-1. Antibody detection. Enzyme immunoassay.** Screening for the presence of antibodies to HIV-1 is often performed by EIA. The antigen used in these tests can be purified HIV-1 particles or HIV-1 recombinant proteins that have been expressed in *E. coli* or in another type of vector. The antigen is attached to a solid phase (such as the plastic bead shown here) and the patient samples are added. Following incubation and washing, an enzyme-labeled antihuman antibody is added. The sample is again incubated and washed. Addition of the substrate results in the formation of a color reaction (first tube on the left) that can be measured with a spectrophotometer. A positive EIA test should be confirmed by Western blot or an immunofluorescent assay.

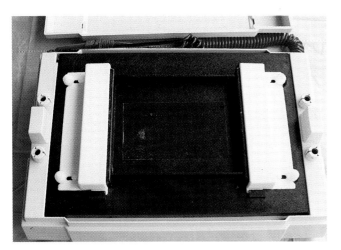

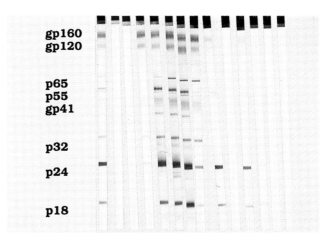

**16-74, 75 Retroviridae. HIV-1. Antibody detection. Western blot test.** Immunoblotting is similar to enzyme immunoassays (EIA). The microorganism of interest, in this case HIV 1, is disrupted using a detergent and heat, and the various viral components (antigens) are separated in a gel by electrophoresis. The antigens on the gel are transferred (blotted) to a nitrocellulose membrane using a special instrument (Figure 16-74, BioRad, Hercules, Calif). Serum from the patient is incubated with strips cut from the membrane. After binding has occurred, enzyme-labeled antihuman globulin and the substrate for the enzyme are added. A colored enzymatic end product is produced in the regions (bands) of the strip where the antibodies from the sample were bound to the antigenic components of the pathogen (Figure 16-75).

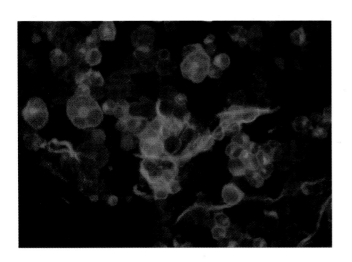

**16-76 Retroviridae. HIV-1. Antibody detection. Immunofluorescent assay (×300).** The substrate for this test consists of a mixture of HIV-1 infected and uninfected H9 cells (a T cell line), which are used to prepare a smear on a microscope slide. The serum to be tested is added and incubated. This is followed by a second incubation with an antihuman immunoglobulin conjugated to fluorescein isothiocyanate. Positive IFA reactions are defined as diffuse cytoplasmic fluorescence, but in certain instances, positive staining patterns may be focal or limited to membrane staining. Nonspecific staining can be adsorbed out using noninfected H9 cells.

# CHAPTER 17 *Immunoserology*

For many infections it is difficult or impossible to isolate an infecting microbe in patient material. Antibodies to specific antigens of pathogens can be used to detect the microbe in such clinical specimens. Alternatively, microbial antigens can be used as targets to detect the presence of a specific antibody response in an infected patient. Unlike culture or direct visualization methods, these immunological techniques may allow determination of past infection and thus immunity to a pathogen. They are not as specific as isolation, however, and the sensitivity is not always as high as desired. If a change in antibody level is necessary for definitive diagnosis, the time to final result may diminish the clinical utility of the procedure. The figures in this section illustrate several standard immunological techniques.

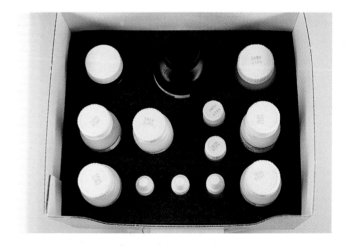

**17-1 Enzyme immunoassays (EIAs) (Abbott Diagnostics, Inc., Chicago, Ill.).** EIAs, or enzyme-linked immunosorbent assays (ELISAs), are frequently used for the detection of antigens or antibodies in clinical samples. Complete kits containing all the necessary reagents are now available for the detection of many microbial antibodies and antigens. Figure 17-1 shows a commercially packaged kit (top view of the bottles, as boxed in a foam support) for the detection of hepatitis C virus antibodies.

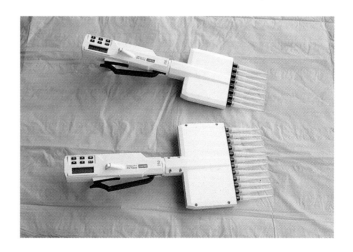

**17-2 Multichannel pipettor (Biohit, Inc., La Jolla, Calif.).** To expedite the testing, multichannel pipettors that allow for the simultaneous delivery or withdrawal of specific amounts of liquids from several samples are used.

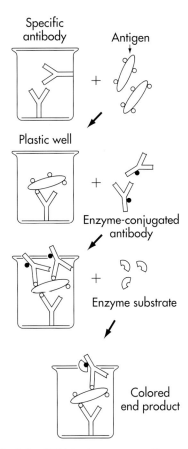

Specific
antibody

Antigen

+

Plastic well

+

Enzyme-conjugated
antibody

+

Enzyme substrate

Colored
end product

**17-3  Direct EIA.** The basic principle of EIA tests uses an antigen or an antibody bound to a solid phase (often a plastic well or a plastic bead) to which the patient sample is added. If the appropriate homologous component is present, antigen-antibody binding occurs. In the direct EIA, a labeled antibody (called a conjugate) against the bound substance is subsequently added to the reaction. The label is usually an enzyme that catalyzes a reaction yielding a colored end product. Addition of the enzyme's substrate results in color development.

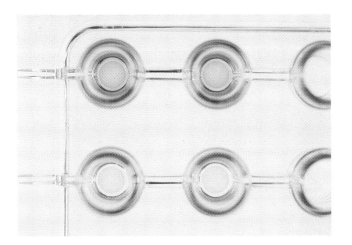

**17-4  Indirect EIA.** For this test, an unlabeled specific antibody is added to the specimen before the second labeled conjugate is added. Thus a single conjugate can be used to detect antibodies of the same Fc type directed against numerous different specific antigens. Figure 17-4 shows a positive reaction in wells on the top row (yellow end product of horseradish peroxidase enzyme and orthophenylenediamine substrate) and negative reactions in the wells on the bottom row. Other conjugates utilizing chemiluminescent, fluorogenic, or radioactive substrates are also in use.

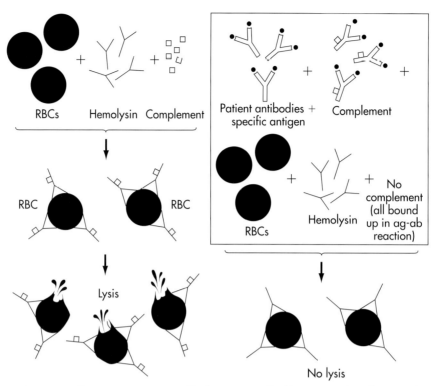

**17-5  Complement fixation method.** In the past, antibodies to certain infectious disease agents, primarily viruses, could be detected only by complement fixation. In this system, an antibody directed against red blood cells (RBC) is able to lyse the RBC only in the presence of complement. The antigen against which the antibodies to be detected have been produced is introduced into the system, along with serum being tested. If the serum contains antibodies, they will bind to the specific antigen, and the subsequent antigen-antibody complexes will bind, or "fix" complement. Without free complement, the antiRBC antibody cannot lyse the RBCs, and they form a button at the bottom of a well in a microtiter plate or a tube.

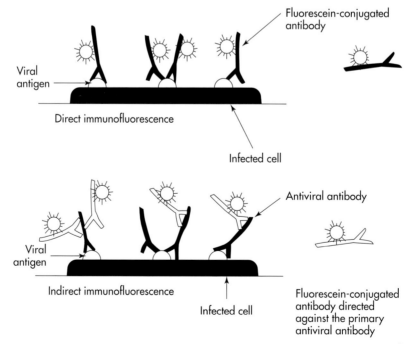

**17-6, 7  Direct and indirect immunofluorescence (IF) methods.** IF methods can be utilized for the detection of specific microbial antigens and antibodies. Direct (Figure 17-6) or indirect (Figure 17-7) approaches can be used.

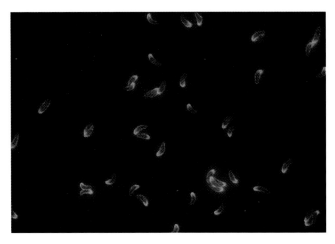

**17-8  Indirect fluorescent antibody method for *Toxoplasma gondii* antibodies.** *T. gondii* cysts on the surface of slides act as the antigen. The serum samples to be tested are layered over the cysts, and the slides are incubated to allow binding of specific anti*Toxoplasma* antibody present in the serum. Subsequently antihuman immunoglobulin conjugated with a fluorescent dye, fluorescein isothiocyanate, is added, and unbound conjugate is washed off. In a positive assay result (Figure 17-8), the microorganisms fluoresce.

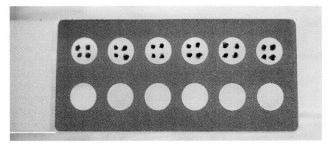

**17-9  Microimmunofluorescence (MIF) test for rickettsial antibodies.** Suspensions of six rickettsial antigens: *Rickettsia rickettsii, R. akari, R. typhi, R. prowazekii,* and *Coxiella burnetii* phase I and II microorganisms are placed as dots on a multiwell glass slide. The top row of wells has been marked with a black pen to demonstrate how several antigen dots can be placed into one well for the MIF test.

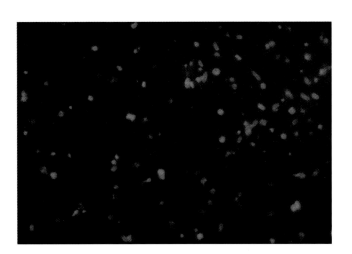

**17-10  Positive MIF test for rickettsial antibodies.** After patient serum and the fluorescein labeled immunoglobulin are added, a positive reaction reveals strongly fluorescing microorganisms of the specific species against which the patient has produced antibody, and may show weakly fluorescent results for the other species.

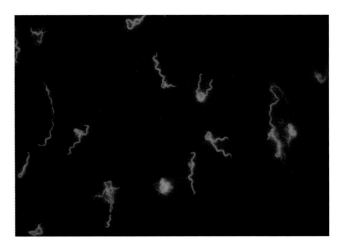

**17-11  Indirect immunofluorescent test for antibodies to *Borrelia burgdorferi*.** *B. burgdorferi,* the spirochetal agent of Lyme disease, is used as substrate. Both IgG and IgM antibodies can be detected.

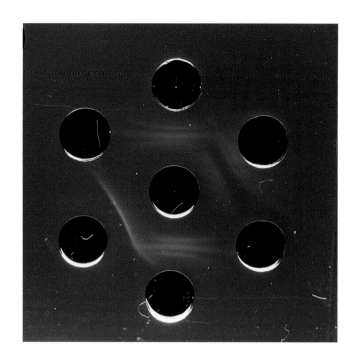

**17-12** *Coccidioides immitis.* **Antibody detection. Passive immunoprecipitation test.** The *C. immitis* antigen is placed in the central well of the gel, and patient and control sera are placed in the six peripheral wells. Immunoprecipitation of the antigen-antibody complex occurs following passive diffusion of the antigens and antibodies toward each other within the gel. To ensure specificity, the positive sample must produce a line of identity with the positive control (e.g., the precipitation line formed by the patient's sample merges with that of the positive control).

**17-13** **Indirect hemagglutination (IHA) test for detection of antibodies to** *Entamoeba histolytica.* In this test, *E. histolytica* antigen is adsorbed onto the surface of tanned human erythrocytes. Sera having specific IgG or IgM antibodies to this microorganism will agglutinate the RBC, which will result in the appearance of a mat in the bottom of the U-shaped wells in a microtiter plate. If the sample does not have antibodies to *E. histolytica*, the RBCs will form a compact cell button (negative control, row 2). In general, patients with extra-intestinal amebiasis develop antibodies 1 to 2 weeks into their symptomatic phase. Positive and negative serum controls and nonsensitized cells should be used in the test to ensure the specificity and sensitivity of the reaction.

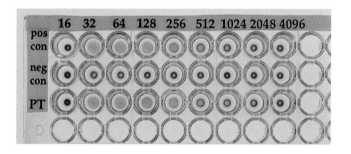

**17-14** **Microhemagglutination assay for the detection of antibodies to** *Treponema pallidum* **(MHA-TP).** This test is used to detect the presence of specific antibodies to *T. pallidum*, present in patients with syphilis. The antigen for the test consists of formalinized tanned sheep RBC sensitized with *T. pallidum* (Nichols strain). The sample is first adsorbed with nonpathogenic Reiter treponemes to remove cross-reactive antibodies. Sensitized sheep RBC are then added. Samples containing antibodies to *T. pallidum* will react with the RBCs, which will form a smooth mat of agglutinated cells at the bottom of the plate (wells 1 through 5, row 1). On the other hand, if there are no antibodies to *T. pallidum*, the unagglutinated RBCs will form a button (row 3).

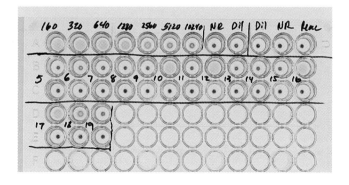

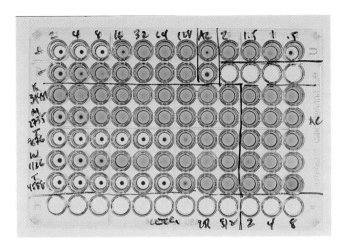

**17-15 Detection of antibodies to *Coccidioides immitis* by the complement fixation (CF) test.** The CF test is based on the ability of complement to lyse RBC in the presence of RBC-specific antibody. Dilutions of the patient sample, *C. immitis* antigen, and guinea pig complement are added to a microtiter plate and allowed to react before a standard amount of sensitized sheep RBC and goat anti-sheep RBC antibody, or hemolysin, is added to the wells. Hemolysis of the sheep RBCs occurs only in those wells that contain free complement, indicating the absence of a specific antigen-antibody reaction (row 3, for example). No hemolysis occurs in the wells where complement fixing antigen-antibody complexes utilized the complement. Thus, samples with antibody will not lyse the RBCs, indicating a positive test (wells 1 through 3, row 1).

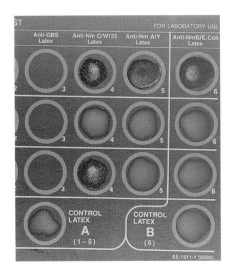

**17-16 Rapid plasma reagin test (RPR).** This test detects the presence of "reagin" antibodies in sera of patients infected with *Treponema pallidum*. It is thought that "reagin" is an antibody developed against tissue lipids. *T. pallidum* damages the tissue of the host causing lipoidal fractions to combine with spirochetal proteins, which subsequently stimulate the production of antibodies. Reagin antibodies are not specific for *T. pallidum*, but they can be used in a sensitive screening test, such as RPR. When the "reagin" binds to the RPR antigen, macroscopic flocculation occurs. The antigen consists of cardiolipin, lecithin, and cholesterol bound to charcoal particles. Choline chloride is added to block complement so that it is not necessary to heat-inactivate the sample. Reactive sera show a clumping of the charcoal particles (top row).

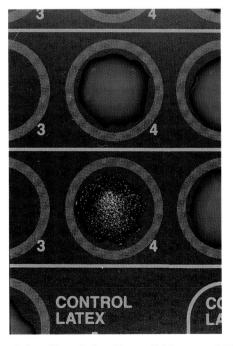

**17-17, 18 Latex particle agglutination test for the detection of *Haemophilus influenzae*, *Streptococcus pneumoniae*, *Neisseria meningitidis*, and group B streptococci (Becton Dickinson Microbiology Systems, Cockeysville, Md.).** Agglutination tests using polystyrene beads coated with specific antibody or antigen are easy and rapid to perform. Antigen-antibody complexes present in a positive test show clumping.

# CHAPTER 18 *Molecular Techniques*

Because clinical specimens often contain very low numbers of an infecting pathogenic microbe, amplification methods can be used to increase the sensitivity of the test and the likelihood of detection. Such methods remove the need to grow the organism in vitro, a slow and variable process. New methods to generate multiple copies of a specific section of nucleic acid of the microorganism being sought allow not only detection of the organism, but detection of specific genetic characteristics, such as a resistance gene. Problems with these techniques include contamination from previously amplified product, inhibition of amplification by specimen components, inability to differentiate viable from nonviable microbes, and interpretation of results. Although the final utility of these methods in clinical microbiology is not yet well-defined, there is no doubt that such techniques will be important elements of the future microbiology laboratory.

**18-1  DNA hybridization.** The DNA hybridization technique is a useful molecular method for the detection and identification of pathogens. The DNA in the specimen is denatured (e.g., the two strands of the DNA molecule are separated using heat or alkali treatment). A labeled single-stranded piece of DNA complementary to a DNA sequence unique to the pathogen being sought (the "probe") is added and hybridizes (binds) to one of the DNA strands of the specimen if it has a complementary sequence (if the pathogen is present). The probe can then be detected by various methods, including enzymatic and radiographic techniques.

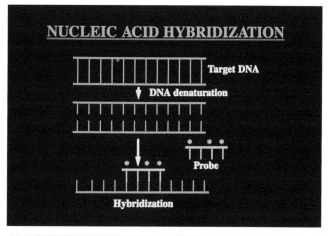

**18-2  Radiolabeled probe detection of herpes virus.** An autoradiogram made from specimens containing herpes simplex virus (HSV-1 or HSV-2) that have been hybridized with $^{32}$P-labeled specific HSV-1 or HSV-2 probes *(left and middle panel)*, or with the two probes simultaneously *(right panel)*.

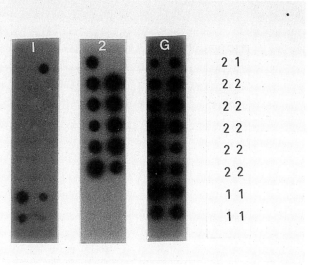

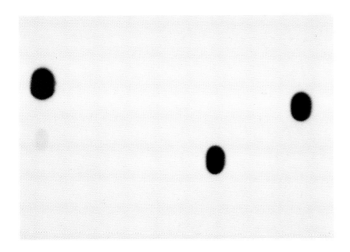

**18-3  DNA hybridization of human papilloma virus probes.** Specimen material treated with radioactive isotope labeled probes for the detection of human papillomaviruses types 6, 11, 16, 31, 33, and 35.

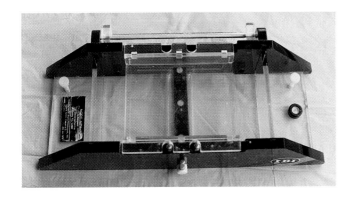

**18-4  Gel apparatus (International Biotechnology, Inc., New Haven, Conn.).** Restriction fragment length polymorphism (RFLP) analysis allows for the detection of genetic differences between organisms. Restriction endonucleases are enzymes that recognize, bind and cleave specific DNA sequences. When the DNA of different organisms is digested with these restriction enzymes, fragments of different sizes may result. After enzyme treatment, DNA fragments are separated on a gel apparatus.

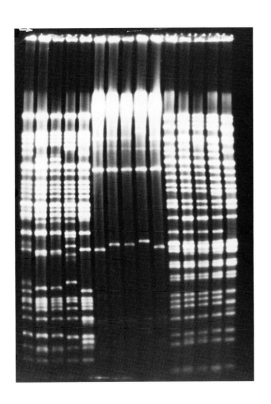

**18-5  Herpes simplex virus DNA restriction patterns.** DNA from five different herpes simplex virus isolates was cleaved with three different restriction endonucleases (five rows per endonuclease), electrophoresed on an agarose gel, and stained with ethidium bromide.

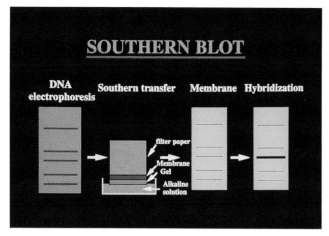

**18-6 Southern blot.** This technique allows for the detection of specific DNA fragments in complex DNA samples. To perform this test, the DNA is first cut with restriction endonucleases. The different size DNA fragments are then separated in a gel based on their electrophoretic mobility (size and charge). The DNA fragments are subsequently transferred, or blotted, onto a nylon membrane or to a similar flat support matrix. The membrane is then hybridized with a specific labeled probe containing the DNA sequence homologous to the one sought. If that sequence is present in the sample DNA, the labeled probe will hybridize to it, and the specific labeled band will be detected in the membrane.

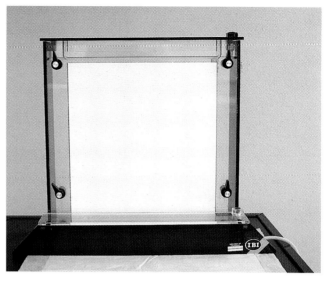

**18-7 DNA sequencing apparatus (International Biotechnology, Inc., New Haven, Conn.).** Four DNA oligonucleotides (short sequences) complementary to one of the strands are synthesized using specific DNA primers. In each of the reactions, a different dideoxynucleoside triphosphate (ddNTP) is randomly incorporated. At the point where a ddNTP, rather than a dNTP, is added, DNA polymerase cannot continue the synthesis, and the strand is truncated. By labeling and separating these fragments based on their length, the DNA sequence of a 300 to 500 base fragment can be determined.

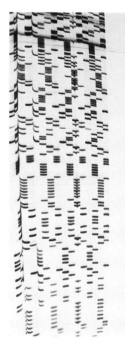

**18-8 Labeled DNA fragments from a sequencing reaction.** This technique allows for the identification of specific microbial isolates and for the determination of the genetic relatedness between different microorganisms.

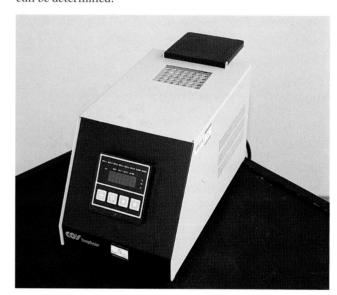

**18-9 Nucleic acid amplification thermocycling instrument (Coy Laboratory Products, Inc., Ann Arbor, Mich.).** The new molecular approaches use biochemical techniques to amplify *in vitro* the nucleic acids of microorganisms of interest in patient specimens. *In vitro* amplification of DNA is mediated by DNA polymerase and amplification of RNA is accomplished after conversion by a reverse transcriptase enzyme to DNA. Several methods for the amplification of nucleic acids require repetitive changes in the temperature of the sample, held in a programmable thermocycling instrument.

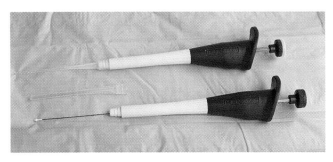

**18-10 Positive displacement pipet used in nucleic amplification tests (Gilson Medical Electronics, Villiers-le-Bel, France).** Amplification methods can result in the production of billions of copies of the same molecule, all concentrated in a very small sample volume. As a result, it is very easy to cross-contaminate specimens during handling of the samples. In order to avoid cross-contamination during pipeting, positive displacement pipets or pipet tips with special filters are used.

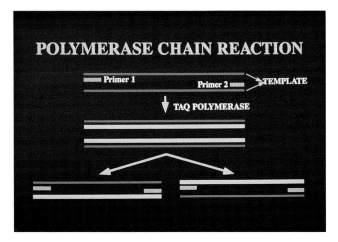

**18-11 Polymerase chain reaction (PCR) basic principle.** This amplification reaction requires two oligonucleotides, 20 to 30 bases in length, complementary to each one of the two strands of a DNA molecule, and separated by approximately 200 to 400 bases in the target molecule. The DNA in the specimen is first denatured by heat, and the oligonucleotides are added to hybridize to their complementary strands. Addition of a DNA polymerase (Taq) that copies the two original strands using the oligonucleotides as primers completes the cycle. The cycle is repeated 30 to 40 times until enough copies of the target DNA can be detected.

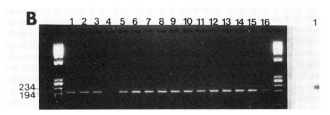

**18-12 PCR reaction products on agarose gel.** The amplified DNA strands in the PCR reaction mixture are separated electrophoretically and stained with ethidium bromide for visualization.

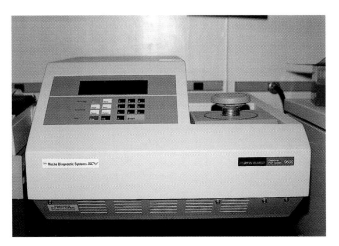

**18-13 Automated PCR instrument (Perkin Elmer, Norwalk, Conn.).** The system includes a thermocycler and an EIA reader to perform and read the result of a PCR that uses an enzyme-labeled detection system.

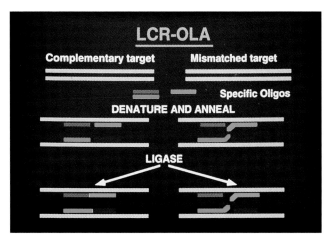

**18-14 Ligase chain reaction (LCR) or oligonucleotide ligation amplification (OLA).** This reaction relies on the enzymatic activity of a DNA ligase to amplify the target nucleic acid. In the LCR, two oligonucleotides homologous to adjacent sequences on the target DNA are joined together by the ligase only when their ends are brought into close proximity by hybridization to the template DNA. Once the ligase has connected the two oligonucleotides, the product of the ligation is denatured from the target DNA so that both the target DNA and the ligated primers can serve again as templates for amplification.

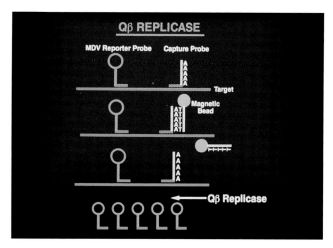

**18-15  Principle of Qβ replicase amplification system.** In the Qβ system, the enzyme Qβ replicase amplifies the signal of the probe and not the target nucleic acid itself. The probe is an RNA molecule known as the midivariant (MDV-1) and a specific RNA fragment corresponding to a complementary piece of RNA or DNA in the organism to be detected. The probe RNA binds to the complementary target, and after removing the unbound MDV-1 molecules, the Qβ replicase is added to replicate the RNA probe.

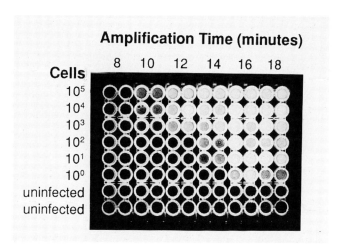

**18-16  Qβ amplification for HIV-1 infected cells detected by fluorescent label.** Very low numbers of HIV-1 infected cells can be detected with this method. (From Pritchard CG, Stefano JE: *Detection of viral nucleic acids by Qβ amplification.* In Medical Virology 10: de la Maza LM and Peterson EM, editors, New York, 1991, Plenum Press.)

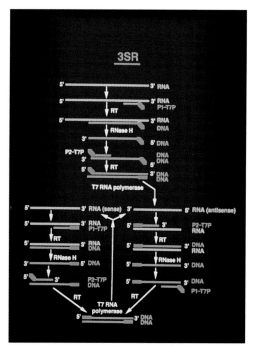

**18-17  Self-sustained sequence replication (3SR).** The avian myoblastosis virus (AMV) reverse transcriptase, the T7 bacteriophage RNA polymerase, and RNase H are utilized in the isothermic amplification of target nucleic acid. The promoter sequence for the T7 RNA polymerase and a region complementary to the target sequence are included in the reaction to allow the polymerase to amplify the target and to provide specificity. The RNase denatures the RNA complement of the RNA-DNA intermediate formed during each amplification phase, allowing sequential amplification to proceed without further high temperature denaturation.

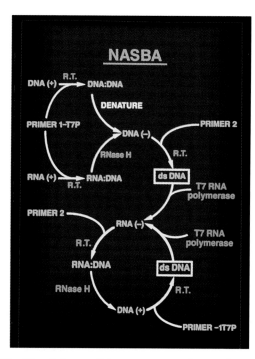

**18-18  Nucleic acid sequence-based amplification (NASBA) method.** Using components similar to those described for 3SR, this system also amplifies nucleic acids at room temperature.

# Index

## A

A 549 cells, *186*

*Absidia*, structure of, *124*

*Absidia corymbifera*
    lactophenol cotton blue preparations of, *125*
    on Sabouraud's dextrose agar, *125*

*Acanthamoeba*, cysts of, *160*

Acid fast stain, Kinyon's, *95*

*Acinetobacter*, *72*

*Acinetobacter baumanii* on MacConkey agar, *86*

*Acinetobacter calcoacetious* var. *anitratus* on MacConkey agar, *86*

*Actinobacillus*, Gram stain of, *29*

*Actinomyces*
    colonies of, *55*
    Gomori methenamine silver stain of, *55*

*Actinomyces israelii*, biochemical identification of, *55*

Adenoviridae, *179–180*

Adenovirus
    antibody detection of, *180*
    culture identification of, with fluorescent stain, *180*
    cytopathic effect of, *179*
    direct fluorescent assay of, *179*
    electron microscopy, negative-stain, *180*
    transmission electron microscopy of, *180*

Adhesive tape technique, fungi, *144*

*Aerococcus*, *37*
    Gram stain of, *26*

Agar disk diffusion method; *see* Disk diffusion method

Agar plates
    contaminated, *5*
    inoculation of, *20–21*

*Aloiococcus*, *37*

*Alternaria*, lactophenol cotton blue preparation of, *119*

Amebae, *146–149*

Amino acid hydrolysis reactions
    of *Nocardia asteroides*, *54*
    of *Nocardia brasiliensis*, *54*
    of *Streptomyces*, *54*

Anaerobes, *88–94*
    media, *22*
    holding jar, *22*
    identification by antimicrobial disks of, *90*
    jar system, *22*
    pouch, *22*

*Ancylostoma duodenale*, egg of, *163*

Antibody detection, *194–199*

Antimicrobial susceptibility testing, *107–112*
    automated, *111*
    broth microdilution, *110*
    disk diffusion, *107, 108*
    E test, *109, 110*

API 20 E strip
    characteristics reactions to, *69*

API 20C clinical yeast system, *145*

API Quad-FERM+ for identifying *Neisseria*, *74*

*Arcanobacterium*, *46*

*Arcanobacterium haemolyticum*, colonies of, *51*

*Ascaris lumbricoides*
    fertile egg of, in feces, *161*
    infertile egg of, in feces, *161*

*Aspergillus*, Gram stain of, *31*
    structure diagram, *119*

*Aspergillus flavus*
    lactophenol cotton blue preparation of, *120*
    on sheep blood agar, *120*

*Aspergillus fumigatus*
    Gram stain of, *120*
    lactophenol cotton blue or calcofluor white preparations of, *121*
    morphology of, *119*
    on sheep blood agar, *120*

*Aspergillus niger*
    lactophenol cotton blue preparation of, *121*
    morphology of, *119*
    on Sabouraud's dextrose agar, *121*

*Aspergillus terreus*
    lactophenol cotton blue preparation of, *122*
    on Sabouraud's dextrose agar, *122*

*Aspergillus versicolor*
    lactophenol cotton blue preparation of, *122*
    morphology of, *119*
    on Sabouraud's dextrose agar, *122*

Auramine fluorescent stain, *95*

Autoclave, *6*

## B

*Babesia microti*, blood stain of, *158*

Bacille Calmette-Guérin vaccine, niacin accumulation testing of, *101*

*Bacillus*
    colonies of, *46, 47*
    egg yolk agar, *47*
    gelatin hydrolysis test for, *47*
    Gram stain, *27, 46*

*Bacillus subtilis*, colonies of, *46*

Bacitracin susceptibility test, *34, 39*

BACTEC blood culture bottles, *13, 23*

Bacteroides bile esculin agar
    *Bacteroides fragilis* on, *88, 91*
    *Prevotella melaninogenica* on, *91*

*Bacteroides fragilis*
    on Bacteroides bile esculin agar (BBE), *88, 91*
    on Brucella blood agar, *88, 90*
    Gram stain, *90*
    identification of, *90*

*Bacteroides urealyticus*, identification of, 90

*Balantidium coli*
cyst of, in feces, 151
trophozoites of, in feces, 151

Bay agar, 53

Beta-lactamase
cefinase for detecting production of, 112
positive test for, 112

Bile esculin slant, 44
of *Enterococcus*, 45

Bile solubility test for *Streptococcus pneumoniae*, 42

Bio-Bag Environmental System, 11

Biological safety cabinet, 6, 7

BioMerieux Vitek colorimeter, 111

*Bipolaris*
germ tube preparation of, 127
lactophenol cotton blue preparation of, 127

*Blastocystis hominis* in feces, 149

*Blastomyces dermatitidis*
colonies of, 113
Gomori methenamine silver stain, 114
lactophenol cotton-blue, preparation of, 113
mycelial phase of, 113
yeast form of, in lung tissue, 114

Blood culture bottles, 12, 13, 23, 24

Blood specimens
collection of, 12, 13

*Bordetella bronchiseptica*
on sheep blood agar, 76
urea identification of, 77

*Bordetella pertussis*
recovery of, 23
specimen collection of, 10

*Bordetella versus Pasteurella*, 76

*Borrelia* sp., Gram stain, 30

*Borrelia burgdorferi*, indirect immunofluorescent test for
antibodies to, 197
Gram stain, 30

*Botryomyces caespitosus* in chromoblastomycosis, 129

Bottles
roller, 178
spinner, 178

*Branhamella* (see *Moraxella*)

Broth microdilution method, 110

*Brucella*, 72
on chocolate agar, 77
Gram stain of, 29, 76
on sheep blood agar, 77

*Burkholderia* (*Pseudomonas*) *cepacia* on MacConkey agar, 87

## C

Caliciviridae, 181

Calicivirus, electron microscopy, negative stain of, in feces, 181

CAMP test
for group B streptococci, 40
for *Clostridium perfringens*, 93

*Campylobacter*, 72
Gram stain of, 30, 80
nalidixic acid susceptibility, 80
recovery of, 23
on TSI slant, 80

*Campylobacter jejuni*
nalidixic acid susceptibility testing for, 80
on TSI slant with lead acetate strip, 80

*Candida*, Gram stain of, 31

*Candida albicans*
on corn meal agar with trypan blue, 123
germ tube test for, with calcofluor white, 123
Gram stain of blood culture of, 123
on sheep blood agar, 122

*Candida glabrata* (see *Torulopsis glabrata*)

*Candida tropicalis*, Gram stain of blood culture of, 123

*Capnocytophaga*, 72
on chocolate agar, 79
on sheep blood agar, 79

*Cardiobacterium*, Gram stain of, 29

Catalase test, 33

Cefinase, detection of beta-lactamase production by, 112

Centrifuge tubes, safety of, 7, 8

Cestodes, 146, 169–173

Charcot-Leyden crystals *versus* parasites in stool, 175

*Chilomastix mesnili*
cyst of, in feces, 151
trophozoite of, in feces, 150

*Chlamydia*, specimen collection of, 10
transport medium, 11

*Chlamydia pneumoniae*
shell vial culture of, 103
transmission electron microscopy of, 104

*Chlamydia psittaci*, shell vial culture of, 103

*Chlamydia trachomatis*
collection kit, 10
direct antigen detection of, 103
direct antigen test of, 181
direct fluorescent assay of, 102
shell vial culture of, 103
transmission electron microscopy of, 104

Chloramphenicol, susceptibility testing of, 109, 110

Chromoblastomycosis
fungi associated with, 129
Gomori's methenamine silver stain of, 129

Ciliates, 150–151

Citrate, utilization of, 60, 64

CIT/RHAM medium, reactions to, 64

*Cladosporium*, 128

*Cladosporium carrionii*
in chromoblastomycosis, 129
lactophenol cotton blue preparation of, 127
on Sabouraud's dextrose agar, 127

Clindamycin, susceptibility testing of, 109

*Clonorchis sinensis*
adult, 167
eggs of, 167

*Clostridium*
  on egg yolk agar, *89*
  Gram stain of, *93*
  identification of, *90*
*Clostridium difficile*
  on Brucella blood agar, *94*
  cytotoxin cell culture assay for, with MRC-5 cells, *102*
  on egg yolk agar, *94*
*Clostridium paraputrificum*, Gram stain of, *94*
*Clostridium perfringens*
  on Brucella blood agar, *93*
  on egg yolk agar, *93, 94*
  reverse CAMP test for, *93*
*Clostridium tertium* on Brucella blood agar, *94*
*Clostridium tetani*
  on Brucella blood agar, *94*
  Gram stain of, *27*
Clothing, protective, *1, 2, 3, 4*
Coagulase test, *Staphylococcus* differentiation with, 34
  slide test, *34*
  tube test, *34*
Coats, laboratory, *3*
Coccidia, *152–153*
*Coccidioides immitis*
  arthroconidia, *155*
  complement fixation test for detecting antibodies to, *199*
  lactophenol cotton-blue preparation of, *115*
  on Gomori's methenamine silver preparation, *115*
  passive immunoprecipitation test for detecting antibodies to, *198*
  on Sabouraud's dextrose agar, *114*
  wet mount and calcofluor white preparations of, *114*
Complement fixation test, *196*
  for detecting antibodies to *Coccidioides immitis*, *199*
Coronaviridae, *181*
Container
  puncture-proof, *5*
  safety bucket, *7*
  mailing, *8*
Coronavirus, electron microscopy, negative stain of, in feces, *181*
*Corynebacterium*, *46*
  Gram stain of, *27, 48*
*Corynebacterium diphtheriae*, colonies of, *48, 49*
  Loeffler's methylene blue stain, *49*
  Tinsdale agar, *49*
*Corynebacterium jeikelum*, colonies of, *48*
*Cryptococcus neoformans*
  on chocolate agar, *115*
  differential identification of, *115*
  India ink and Gram stain of, *31, 116*
  mixed culture of, with *Histoplasma capsulatum*, *118*
  urease test for, *116*
*Cryptosporidium parvum*, oocysts of, in feces, *153*
CTA (see cystine-trypticase agar)
Culture(s)
  aerobic
    collection and transport of, *9*
    incubation of, *21*

anaerobic
  collection and transport of, *11*
  incubation of, *21*
  media, *16, 23*
Cysticercus, *Taenia solium* in, *170*
Cystine-trypticase agar (CTA) for identifying *Neisseria* species, *73*
Cytomegalovirus, *183*
  antibody detection of, *185*
  cytopathic effect of, *184*
  hemotoxylin and eosin, *185*
  horseradish peroxidase, *185*
  in kidney and lung, *185*
  shell vial of, with immunofluorescent stain, *184*
Cytotoxin cell culture assay with MRC-5 cells for *Clostridium difficile*, *102*

**D**

Decarboxylase-dihydrolase test, *62*
Diarrhea, antibiotic-associated, *102*
*Dientamoeba fragilis*, trophozoite of, in feces, *150*
*Diphyllobothrium latum*, egg of, in feces, *169*
Diplococci, gram-positive, *26*
*Dipylidium caninum*
  proglottids of, *172*
  scolex of, *172*
Disinfection, *4*
Disk diffusion method, 107, 108
  with *Escherichia coli* ATCC 25922, *108*
  with *Pseudomonas aeruginosa* ATCC 27853, *109*
  with resistant strain of *Pseudomonas aeruginosa*, *109*
  with *Staphylococcus aureus* ATCC 25923, *108*
  with *Streptococcus pneumoniae*, *109*
Disposal, waste, *4, 5*
DNA hybridization, *200*
  of herpes simplex virus, *200*
  of human papilloma virus, *201*
DNA probes, fungi, *145*
DNA restriction patterns in herpes simplex virus, *201*
DNA sequencing, *202*
DNase agar, *86*

**E**

E test method for *Streptococcus pneumoniae*, *109, 110*
*Echinococcus granulosus*
  adult worm, *172*
  eggs of, *173*
  hydatid sand, *173*
  hydatid cyst in liver, *173*
Echovirus 11, cytopathic effect of, in MRC-5 cells, *191*
EIA (see enzyme immunoassay)
*Eikenella*, *72*
  Gram stain of, *29*
*Eikenella corrodens* on sheep blood agar, *78*
Electron microscopy
  of *Adenovirus*, *180*
  of *Calicivirus*, *181*
  of *Chlamydia pneumonia*, *104*

Electron microscopy *(continued)*
    of *Chlamydia trachomatis*, *104*
    of *Coronavirus*, *181*
    of Herpes virus, *183*
    of HIV-1, *192*
    of *Rotavirus*, *192*
    of *Ureaplasma urealyticum*, *106*
    of *Vaccinia virus*, *192*
ELISA (see enzyme immunoassays)
Endocarditis, agents of, *29*
*Endolimax nana*
    cyst of, in feces, *149*
    trophozoite of, in feces, *148*
*Entamoeba coli*
    cyst of, in feces, *148*
    trophozoite of, in feces, *148*
*Entamoeba hartmanni*
    cyst of, in feces, *148*
    trophozoites of, in feces, *147*
*Entamoeba histolytica*
    cysts of, in feces, *147*
    indirect hemagglutination test for detecting antibodies to, *198*
    trophozoites of
        in liver, *147*
        in feces, *146*
*Enterobacter aerogenes*, characteristic reactions of, in API 20 E strips, *68, 69*
*Enterobacter cloacae*, characteristic reactions of, in API 20 E strips, *68*
Enterobacteriaceae, 56–71
    characteristics of, *56*
    citrate utilization test for, *60*
    decarboxylase-dihydrolase test for, *62*
    Gram stain, *30*
    on Hektoen enteric agar, *58*
    indole spot test for, *59*
    on MacConkey agar, *58*
    methyl red-Voges-Proskauer test for, *59*
    ONPG test for, *59*
    oxidase spot test for, *59*
    PAD test for, *61*
    phenylalanine deaminase test for, *60*
    rapid spot test identification of, *58*
    on sheep blood agar, *56*
    triple sugar iron test for, *62*
    urea test for, *61*
    urease test for, *61*
*Enterobius vermicularis*
    adult female and male, *161*
    eggs of
        cellophane tape preparation of, *162*
        in feces, *162*
*Enterococcus*, *37, 44*
    bile esculin agar, *45*
    colonies of, *45*
    NaCl broth, 6.5%, *45*
Enzyme immunoassays (EIA), *194*
    direct, *195*
    indirect, *195*
*Epidermophyton floccosum*
    lactophenol cotton blue preparation of, *132*
    on Sabouraud's dextrose agar, *132*

Epithelial cells, ciliated columnar, *versus* parasites, in feces, *175*
Epstein-Barr virus, *183*
    commercial particle agglutination test for serological diagnosis of, *186*
    heterophile antibody, *186*
    immunofluorescent tests for antibodies to nuclear antigens of, *187*
    immunofluorescent tests for antibodies to early and structural antigens of, *187*
*Erysipelothrix*, 46
*Erysipelothrix rhusiopathiae* on TSI agar, *50*
    colonies of, *50*
Erythromycin, susceptibility testing of, *109*
*Escherichia coli*
    characteristic reactions of, *67*
        in API 20 E strip, *68*
    Gram stain of, *30*
    on MacConkey agar, *57*
    in Micro-ID, *67*
    on sheep blood agar, *57*
Esculin hydrolysis test, *48*
*Exophiala (Wangiella) dermatitidis*, lactophenol cotton blue preparation of, *128*
*Exophiala jeanselmei*
    lactophenol cotton blue preparation of, *128*
    on Sabouraud's dextrose agar, *128*
*Exserohilum*, lactophenol cotton blue preparation of, *128*
Eye wear, *2*

**F**

Face mask
    conditions requiring, *2*
    improperly fitted, *3*
Face shield, *3*
*Fasciola hepatica*, egg of, in feces, *167*
Filaria, 165–166
Flagellates, 150–151
Flasks, tissue culture, *177*
Flatworms; *see* Trematodes
*Flavobacterium*, 72
*Flavobacterium meningosepticum* on sheep blood agar, *86*
*Fonsecaea compacta* in chromoblastomycosis, *129*
*Fonsecaea pedrosoi*
    in chromoblastomycosis, *129*
    lactophenol cotton blue preparation of, *129*
Fungi; *see also* Mycology; specific fungi
    classification and characteristics of, *113*
    identification of, *113*
*Fusarium*
    lactophenol cotton blue preparation of, *140*
    on potato dextrose agar, *140*
*Fusobacterium*
    egg yolk agar for identifying, *89*
    Gram stain of, *30*
    identification of, *90*
    spot indole disk test of, *89*
*Fusobacterium nucleatum*
    on Brucella blood agar, *92*
    Gram stain of, *30, 92*

# G

Gamma hemolysis, *38*

*Gardnerella*, 46

*Gardnerella vaginalis*
colonies of, *50*
Gram stain of, *50*
hippurate hydrolysis test for, *50*

GasPak
anaerobic jar system, *22*
anaerobic pouch, *23*

Gelatin hydrolysis test, *47*

*Gemella*, 37

*Geotrichum* on corn meal agar with trypan blue, *124*

*Giardia lamblia*
cyst of, in feces, *150*
trophozoite of, in feces, *150*

*Globicatella*, 37

Gloves, removal and disposal of, *1, 2*

Goggles, conditions requiring, *2*

Gram stain, *25–31*
preparation of, *24*

*Graphium conidia*, lactophenol cotton blue stain of, *130*

# H

HACEK, Gram stain of, *29*

*Haemophilus*, 72
Gram stain of, *29, 30*

*Haemophilus aphrophilus*, Minitek sugar identification of, *76*

*Haemophilus influenzae*
on chocolate agar, *74*
Latex particle agglutination test for detecting, *199*
porphyrin production test for, *75*
on X and V strips, *75*
satelliting, *75*

*Haemophilus parainfluenzae*
on chocolate agar, *75*
Minitek sugar identification of, *76*

Hektoen enteric agar, Enterobacteriaceae on, *58*

Helminths, classification of, *146*

Hemolysis
alpha, *37*
gamma, *38*

Hepatitis C, EIA detection of, *194*

Herpes simplex virus
antibody detection of, *184*
cervical swab of, *182*
cytopathic effect of, *182*
direct antigen test of, *181*
direct immunofluorescent assay of, *182*
DNA probe, *200*
DNA restriction patterns in, *201*
horseradish peroxidase stain, *182*
shell vial culture of, *183*
skin lesions with, *181*
transmission electron microscopy of, *183*

Herpes virus
collection kit, *10*
radiolabeled probe detection of, *200*
specimens of, *10*

Herpesviridae, *181–186*

Heterophile antibody, *186*

Hippurate hydrolysis test, *40*
for *Gardnerella vaginalis*, *50*
for group B streptococci, *40*
for *Listeria monocytogenes*, *48*

*Histoplasma capsulatum*
on buffy coat preparation (Wright's stain), *117*
colonies of, *116*
differential identification of, *115*
on direct bone marrow preparation stained with calcofluor white, *117*
lactophenol cotton blue stained colonies of, *117*
lung section showing, with Gomori's methenamine silver, *117*
mixed culture of, with *Cryptococcus neoformans*, *118*
yeast form of, *116*

Homogenization of specimens, *17*

Hookworm, egg of, *163*

Human immunodeficiency virus type 1
antibody detection of
with enzyme immunoassay, *193*
with immunofluorescent assay, *193*
with Western blot testing, *193*
positive Qβ amplification for, *204*
transmission electron microscopy, *192*

Human papilloma virus, DNA hybridization of, *201*

*Hymenolepis diminuta*, egg of, in feces, *172*

*Hymenolepis nana*, egg of, in feces, *171*

# I

Immunofluorescence, direct and indirect, *196*

Immunoserology, *194–199*

Indole spot test, *59*
for anaerobes, *89*

Influenza A virus
African green monkey kidney cell isolation of, *188*
direct fluorescent assay of, *187*
hemadsorption, *188*

Influenza virus
antibody detection of, *188*
shell vial culture of, *188*

Inoculum
preparation of, *107*
turbidity meter for adjusting, *107*

Interstate Shipment of Etiologic Agents, *8*

*Iodamoeba bütschlii*
cyst of, in feces, *149*
trophozoite of, in feces, *149*

Iron uptake test, *101*

Isolatorlysis-centrifugation blood culture system, *12*

*Isospora belli*, cyst of, in feces, *152*

# J

JC virus in progressive multifocal leukoencephalopathy, brain tissue section of, *189*

Jembec plate, *11*

# K

*Kingella,* 72
    Gram stain of, *29*

*Kingella kingae* on sheep blood agar, *78, 79*

Kinyoun acid-fast stain, *95*
    modified, for *Nocardia, 53*
    modified, for *Rhodococcus equi, 52*

*Klebsiella oxytoca,* characteristic reactions of, to API 20 E strips, *69*

*Klebsiella pneumoniae*
    on MacConkey agar, *57*
    urease test for, *61*

*Klebsiella versus Rhodococcus equi, 51*

# L

Laboratory coats, *3*

Laboratory safety, 1–8
    and biological safety cabinets, *6, 7*
    and disinfection, waste disposal, and sterilization, *4, 5, 6*
    mailing containers and, *8*
    miscellaneous practices and, *7, 8*
    and protective clothing and equipment, 1, 2, 3, 4

Lactobacilli, Gram stain of, *27*

*Lactobacillus, 46*
    colonies of, *49*
    Gram stain of, in vaginal secretions, *49*

*Lactococcus, 37, 44*

Latex particle agglutination test for detecting *H. influenzae, S. pneumoniae, N. meningitidis,* and group B streptococci, *199*

LCR (ligase chain reaction)

Lead acetate strip, *Campylobacter jejuni* on, *80*

*Legionella pneumophila* on buffered charcoal-yeast extract agar, *87*

*Leishmania*
    amastigotes of, *159*
    promastigotes of, *159*

*Leuconostoc, 37, 44*
    colonies of, *45*

Leukoencephalopathy, progressive multifocal, JC virus in, *189*

Ligase chain reaction (LCR), *203*

Liquid nitrogen tanks, *179*

*Listeria, 46*

*Listeria monocytogenes*
    colonies of, *47*
    esculin hydrolysis test for, *48*
    Gram stain of, *27*
    hippurate hydrolysis, *48*

Liver, *Echinococcus granulosus* in, *173*

*Loa loa,* microfilariae of, *165*

Loeffler methylene blue stain of *C. diphtheriae, 49*

# M

MRVP broth test (see Methyl red-Voges-Proskauer)

Mailing containers, safety requirements for, 8

Malaria, 155–158
    development of, *155*

*Malassezia furfur*
    Gram stain and calcofluor white preparations of, *133*
    on Sabouraud's dextrose agar, *132*

Mannitol salt agar, *Staphylococcus aureus* differentiation with, *35*

Measles virus
    antibody detection of, with indirect immunofluorescent assay, *190*
    in lung tissue, *190*
    phytohemagglutinin stimulated cord blood mononuclear cell culture of, *189*
    Vero cell culture of, *190*

Methyl red-Voges-Proskauer (MRVP) broth test, *59*

MIC, defined, *107*

Micrococcaceae, 32–36
    morphology of, *32*

*Micrococcus*
    Gram stain of, *33*
    infections due to, *32*
    *versus Staphylococcus, 32*

Microhemagglutination assay for detecting antibodies to *Treponema pallidum, 198*

MICRO-ID strip, *E. coli* reactions to, *67*

Microimmunofluorescence test
    for *Mycoplasma* and *Ureaplasma, 106*
    for rickettsial antibodies, *197*

Microscopes
    brightfield, with epiluminescence, *176*
    inverted, *176*

*Microsporidium,* 152–153
    in feces, *153*

*Microsporum audouinii*
    lactophenol cotton blue preparation of, *133*
    on Sabouraud's dextrose agar, *133*

*Microsporum canis* var. *canis*
    lactophenol cotton blue preparation of, *134*
    on Sabouraud's dextrose agar, *134*

*Microsporum gypseum*
    lactophenol cotton blue preparation of, *135*
    on Sabouraud's dextrose agar, *134*

Minitek sugars for identifying *Haemophilus, 76*

Molds, specimen preparation and identification systems for, 144–145

Molecular techniques, 200–204

Monospot test, *188*

*Moraxella,* 72

*Moraxella (Branhamella) catarrhalis* on sheep blood agar, *73*

*Morganella morganii*
    characteristic reactions of, in API 20 E strips, *70*
    PAD and urea tests for, *61*

MRC-5 cells, *102*

*Mucor*
    Gomori's methenamine silver stain of, *126*
    lactophenol cotton blue preparation of, *126*
    structure of, *124*

Multichannel pipettor, *194*

*Mycobacterium,* 95–101

*Mycobacterium avium*
    on Löwenstein-Jensen agar, *97*
    on Middlebrook 7H11 agar, *97*
    rough colony of, *97*
    smooth colony of, *97*
*Mycobacterium chelonae*
    on chocolate agar, *99*
    colony of, *99*
    on Middlebrook 7H11 agar, *99*
*Mycobacterium fortuitum*
    colony of, *100*
    iron uptake test for differentiating, *101*
    on Löwenstein-Jensen agar, *100*
    on Middlebrook 7H11 agar, *99*
*Mycobacterium gordonae*
    on Löwenstein-Jensen agar, *100*
    on Middlebrook 7H11 agar, *100, 101*
*Mycobacterium kansasii*
    colony of, *98*
    on Löwenstein-Jensen agar, *98*
    on Middlebrook 7H11 agar, *98*
*Mycobacterium simiae*, niacin accumulation testing of, *101*
*Mycobacterium tuberculosis*
    colonies of, *96*
    on Löwenstein-Jensen agar slant, *96*
    on Middlebrook 7H11, *96*
    niacin accumulation testing of, *101*
Mycology, *113–145*
*Mycoplasma*
    antibody detection of, by microimmunofluorescence test, *106*
    characteristics of, *105*
*Mycoplasma hominis* colonies, *105*
Mycoses
    deep-seated, *113–118*
    miscellaneous, *140–143*
    opportunistic, 113, *119–126*
    specimen preparation and identification systems for, *144–145*
    subcutaneous, *127–131*
    superficial, *132–139*
    systemic, 113

## N

Nalidixic acid, *Campylobacter jejuni* susceptibility to, *80*
Nasopharyngeal
    collection system, *10*
    -urogenital swab, *9*
National Committee for Clinical Laboratory Standards, 107
*Necator americanus*
    egg of, *163*
    first-stage rhabditiform larvae of, *163*
Needles, disposal of, *5*
*Neisseria*, 72
    API Quad-FERM+ identification of, *74*
    carbohydrate utilization identification of, *73*
    Gram stain of, *29, 72*
    *Neisseria/Haemophilus* identification card for identifying, *74*
*Neisseria gonorrhoeae*
    Gram stain of, *29*
    on modified Thayer-Martin agar, *73*
    recovery of, *23*
    specimen collection of, *9*

*Neisseria meningitidis*
    on chocolate agar, *72*
    Gram stain of, *29*
    latex particle agglutination test for detecting, *199*
    on sheep blood agar, *73*
*Neisseria/Haemophilus* identification (NHI) card for identifying *Neisseria*, 74
Nematodes, 146, *161–166*
    intestinal, *161–164*
    tissue, *164–166*
NHI card (see *Neisseria/Haemophilus* identification card)
Niacin accumulation test, *101*
Nitrate test, *77*
    disk test, *89*
*Nocardia*
    biochemical reactions for identifying, *54*
    colonies of, *53*
    Gram stain of, *53*
    on Bay agar, *53*
*Nocardia asteroides*
    amino acid hydrolysis reactions of, *54*
    colonies of, *53*
*Nocardia brasiliensis*, amino acid hydrolysis reactions of, *54*
Novobiocin susceptibility test, *36*
Nucleic acid amplification thermocycling instrument, *202*
Nucleic acid sequence-based amplification method, *204*
Nucleic amplification tests, positive displacement pipette for, *203*

## O

ONPG test (see O-nitrophenyl-β-D-galactosidase test)
Occupational Safety and Health Act, safety provisions of, 1
*Oerskovia*, 46
    colonies of, *52*
    Gram stain of, *28*
Oligonucleotide ligation amplification, *203*
*Onchocerca volvulus*, microfilaria, *166*
O-nitrophenyl-β-D-galactosidase (ONPG) test, *59*
Optochin susceptibility test
    for *Streptococcus pneumoniae*, *42*
    of viridans streptococci, *43*
Orthomyxoviridae, *187–189*
OSHA; *see* Occupational Safety and Health Act
Oxacillin
    screen plate, *35*
    *Staphylococcus aureus* resistance to, detection of, *35*
    susceptibility testing of, *109*
Oxidase spot test, *59*
Oxidative-fermentative medium, *33, 82*
    glucose oxidation in, *33*
    glucose fermentation in, *33*

## P

PAD test (see phenylalanine deaminase test)
*Paecilomyces variotti*
    lactophenol cotton blue preparation of, *141*
    on Sabouraud's dextrose agar, *141*

Papovaviridae, *189*

*Paracoccidioides brasiliensis*
in adrenal tissue, stained with Gomori's methenamine silver, *118*
differential identification of, *115*
stained with lactophenol cotton blue, *118*

*Paragonimus westermani*, egg of, in feces, *168*

Parainfluenza 3 and 4 viruses, immunofluorescent staining of, *189*

Paramyxoviridae, *189–191*

Para-Pak Parasitology Collection Kit, *12*

Parasites, specimen collection of, *12*

Parasitology, *146–175*

*Pasteurella*, *72*

*Pasteurella multocida* on sheep blood agar, *78*

PCR (polymerase chain reaction)

*Pediococcus*, *37*
colonies of, *44*
vancomycin susceptibility testing of, *44*

Penicillin
*Streptococcus pneumoniae* resistance to, *43*

*Penicillium*
diagram of, *141*
on Sabouraud's dextrose agar, *142*
stained with calcofluor white, *142*

*Penicillium marneffei*
lactophenol cotton blue and calcofluor white preparations of, *143*
on Sabouraud's dextrose agar, *142*

*Peptostreptococcus*, spot indole disk test of, *89*

*Peptostreptococcus anaerobius* on Brucella blood agar, *92*
identification of, *90*

*Peptostreptococcus magnus*
on Brucella blood agar, *92*
SPS resistance of, *92*

*Peptostreptotoccus anaerobius*, sodium polyanethol sulfonate disk test of, *89*

Personal Protective Devices, *1, 2, 3, 4*

Phenylalanine deaminase (PAD) test, *60, 61*

*Phialophora*, *128*

*Phialophora verrucosa*
in chromoblastomycosis, *129*
lactophenol cotton blue preparation of, *129*

Picornaviridae, *191–192*

Pinworm, *161*

Pipet, positive displacement, *203*

Pipettor, multichannel, *194*

Plant cells *versus* parasites, in feces, *174*

Plantar spiral *versus* parasites in feces, *175*

*Plasmodium falciparum*
gametocyte appearance and, *157*
ring forms of, *155*
thick blood smear of, *155, 157*
trophozoites of, *155*

*Plasmodium malariae*
schizonts and, *157*
trophozoites of, *156*

*Plasmodium ovale*
erythrocyte appearance and, *156*
Schüffner's dots and, *156*
thick blood smear of, *157*

*Plasmodium vivax*
macrogametocytes, *158*
microgametocytes, *158*
*versus P. falciparum*, *156*
Schüffner's dots and, *156*
thick blood smear of, *157*

Plates, multiple well, *177*

*Pneumocystis carinii*
from bronchoalveolar lavage, *154*
from lung biopsy, *154*
in sputum, *153*

Pollen *versus* parasites in feces, *174*

Polymerase chain reaction (PCR)
automated instrument for, *203*
basic principle of, *203*
products of, on agarose gel, *203*

Polymorphonuclear leukocytes, *26, 27*
Gram stain of, *28, 53*
with gram-positive bacilli, *75*
poorly differentiated, *30*

Porphyrin production test for *Haemophilus influenzae*, *75*

*Porphyromonas*, spot indole disk test of, *89*

Positive displacement pipette for nucleic amplification tests, *203*

Poxviridae, *192*

*Prevotella*, spot indole disk test of, *89*
identification of, *90*

*Prevotella melaninogenica*
on Bacteroides bile esculin agar, *91*
on Brucella blood agar, *91*
Gram stain of, *91*

Progressive multifocal leukoencephalopathy, JC virus in, *189*

*Propionibacterium*, spot indole disk test of, *89*

*Proprionibacterium acnes* on Brucella blood agar, *93*

*Proteus*
Gram stain of, *30*
on sheep blood agar, *56*

*Proteus mirabilis*
characteristic reactions of
in API 20 E strips, *69, 70*
PAD and urea tests for, *61*
urease test for, *61*

*Proteus vulgaris*
characteristic reactions of, *66*
to API 20 E strips, *70*
with API 20 E strips, *69*
PAD and urea tests for, *61*

Protozoans, *146–160*
coccidia and microsporidia, *152–153*
flagellates and ciliates, *150–151*
intestinal, *146–149*
in tissue, *153–154*

*Providencia rettgeri*, PAD and urea tests for, *61*

*Pseudallescheria boydii*
on Sabouraud's dextrose agar, *130*
sexual state of, lactophenol cotton blue stain of, *130*

Pseudomonadaceae, 82–86

*Pseudomonas,* 72
    Gram stain of, *30*

*Pseudomonas aeruginosa*
    GNF, urea, and Pseudosel agar for identifying, *84*
    GNF tube identification of, *83*
    on MacConkey agar, *83*
    pigment production by, *83*
    resistant strain of, disk diffusion method for, *109*
    on sheep blood agar, *82*
    on TSI slant, *83*
    Uni-N/F-Tek plate for identifying, *84*

*Pseudomonas aeruginosa* ATCC 27853, disk diffusion method
    for, *109*

*Pseudomonas cepacia,* (see *Burkholderia cepacia*)

*Pseudomonas paucimobilis,* (see *Sphingomonas paucimobilis*)

*Pseudomonas putrefaciens,* (see *Shewanella putrefaciens*)

PYR test, *39*

**Q**

Qβ replicase amplification
    for HIV-1 infected cells detected by fluorescent label, *204*
    principle of, *204*

**R**

Radiolabeled probe for detecting herpesvirus, *200*

Rapid plasma reagin (RPR) test, *199*

Rapid spot test for Enterobacteriaceae, *58*

r/b₂ medium, reactions to, *64*

r/b tube
    for Enterobacteriaceae, *62*
    reactions to, *63*

Reoviridae, *192*

Respiratory syncytial virus
    culture identification of, in MRC-5 cells in shell vial, *191*
    cytopathic effect of, in MRC-5 cells, *191*
    direct fluorescent assay of, *190*

Restriction fragment length polymorphism analysis, *201*

Retroviridae, *192–193*

Rhamnose, fermentation of, *64*

*Rhinocladiella,* *128*

*Rhinocladiella aquaspersa* in chromoblastomycosis, *129*

Rhinovirus, cytopathic effect of, in MRC-5 cells, *192*

*Rhizopus*
    lactophenol cotton blue preparation of, *126*
    structure of, *124*

*Rhodococcus,* 46
    colonies of, *51*
    microscopic appearance of, *52*

*Rhodococcus equi,* classification of, *51*
    acid fast stain, *51*

*Rickettsia,* microimmunofluorescence test for detecting antibod-
    ies to, *197*

Rifampin, susceptibility testing of, *109*

Roller bottles, *178*

Roller drum, *177*

Rotavirus, electron microscopy of, in stool, *192*

Roundworms; *see* Nematodes

RPR (see rapid plasma reagin test)

**S**

Safety; *see* Laboratory safety

Safety cabinet, biological, *6, 7*

Saliva *versus* sputum, *18*

*Salmonella*
    characteristic reactions of, *65*
    on Hektoen enteric agar, *58, 71*
    triple sugar iron agar test for, *62*

*Salmonella enteritidis,* colonial morphology *versus* biochemical
    identification of, *71*

*Salmonella typhi,* characteristic reactions of, *65*

Salt broth, 6.5%, *45*

Samples; *see* Specimens

*Scedosporium apiospermum,* lactophenol cotton blue stain of,
    *130*

*Scedosporium prolificans,* lactophenol cotton blue stain of, *131*

Schüffner's dots, *156*

*Schistosoma haematobium,* egg of, *168*

*Schistosoma japonicum*
    adult male of, *168*
    cercaria, *168*
    egg of, *168*

*Schistosoma mansoni,* egg of, in stool, *169*

Schlichter test, *112*

*Scopulariopsis*
    lactophenol cotton blue preparation of, *143*
    on Sabouraud's dextrose agar, *143*

Self-sustained sequence replication, principle (SSSR), *204*

Septi-Chek biphasic blood culture bottle, *12*

*Serratia marcescens,* characteristic reactions of, with API 20 E
    strips, *69*

*Serratia* on MacConkey agar, *57*

Serum inhibitory titer, *112*

Shell vial, *177*

*Shewanella,* 72

*Shewanella (Pseudomonas) putrefaciens*
    on sheep blood agar, *85*
    TSI reaction of, *85*

*Shigella,* characteristic reactions of, *67*

*Shigella sonnei,* characteristic reactions of, to API 20 E strips, 70

Skin, protection of, *4*

Sleeping sickness, *159–160*

Slide culture method for fungi, *144*

Slides
    preparation of, *19, 20*
    wet, *20*

Smears
    fixing and staining of, *24*
    preparation of, *19*

Sodium chloride test
    6.5%, *45*
    tolerance test, *101*

Sodium polyanethol sulfonate disk test
for *Peptostreptococcus anaerobius*, 89
for *Peptostreptococcus magnus*, 92

Southern blot test, *202*

Specimens
anaerobic
media for, *16*
prereduced, *22*

Specimens *(continued)*
blood, *12, 13*
of *Bordetella pertussis*, *10*
chlamydial, *10*
collection containers for, *9–13*
containers for, *15*
culture of, media for, *16*
discrepancy between microscopic and gross appearances of, *19*
disposal of, *5*
entering into computer system, *14, 15*
of expectorated sputa, *15*
homogenizing of, *17*
inspection of, before inoculation of media, *18*
labeling of, *14*
mailing containers for, *8*
of *Neisseria gonorrhoeae*, *9, 10*
processing of, *14–24*
atmospheric conditions for, *21, 22*
equipment for, *17*
procedure manual for, *16*
rapid direct tests for, *24*
quality of, *18, 19*
in syringes, *21*
transport of, *9*
urethral, collection of, *9*
viral, *10, 11*

*Sphingomonas*, *72*
on sheep blood agar, *84*

*Sphingomonas (Pseudomonas) paucimobilis* on sheep blood agar, *84*

Spinner bottles, *178*

*Sporothrix schenckii*
lactophenol cotton blue preparation of, *131*
on potato dextrose agar, *131*

Spot indole disk test, uses of, *89*

Sputum
*versus* saliva, *18*
specimens of, *15, 19*

Squamous epithelial cells, vaginal, *27*

SSSR (see self-sustained sequence replication)

*Staphylococcus saprophyticus*, colonial morphology of, *36*

*Staphylococcus*
coagulase-negative, *32*
infections due to, *32*
*versus Micrococcus*, *33*
*versus Streptococcus*, *75*
with *Streptococcus*, *27*
susceptibility testing for, *107*
in upper respiratory tract, *38*

*Staphylococcus aureus*, *32*
antimicrobial susceptibility testing of, *35*
colonies of, *32*
differentiation of
by coagulase test, *34*

with mannitol salt agar, *35*
Gram stain of, *26*
methicillin (and oxacillin)-resistant, detection of, *35*

*Staphylococcus saprophyticus*, novobiocin susceptibility differential testing of, *36*

*Stenotrophomonas*, *72*

*Stenotrophomonas (Xanthomonas) maltophilia*
on sheep blood agar, *85*
Uni-N/-Tek for identifying, *85*

Sterilization, *6*

*Stomatococcus*
Gram stain of, *26*
infections due to, *32*

Streptococcaceae, *37–45*

*Streptococcus*, *37*
alpha-hemolytic, *37*
beta-hemolytic, *37*
gamma hemolysis, *37*
Gram stain, *27*
group A, *38, 39*
PYR test of, *39*
group A beta-hemolytic, bacitracin susceptibility test of, *39*
group B, *40*
CAMP test for, *40*
hippurate hydrolysis test of, *40*
latex particle agglutination test for detecting, *199*
group D, bile esculin slant and NaCl broth testing of, *45*
nonhemolytic, *38*
*versus Staphylococcus*, *75*
with *Staphylococcus*, *27*
in vaginal secretions, *40*
viridans
conventional biochemical reaction testing of, *43*
Gram stain of, *43*
optochin susceptibility test of, *43*

*Streptococcus bovis*, bile esculin slant testing of, *44*

*Streptococcus pneumoniae*
antimicrobial susceptibility testing of, *43*
bile solubility test for, *42*
colonies of, *41, 42*
E test method for, *109, 110*
Gram stain of, *41*
latex particle agglutination test for detecting, *199*
optochin susceptibility test for, *42*
secondary test battery for, *109*

*Streptococcus pyogenes*, colonies of, *51*

*Streptomyces*
amino acid hydrolysis reactions of, *54*
Gram stain of, *55*

*Strongyloides stercoralis*
filariform larvae of, *164*
first-stage rhabditiform larvae of, *163, 164*

Swab, nasopharyngeal-urogenital, *9*

Syringes, specimens in, *21*


**T**

*Taenia*, eggs of, *171*

*Taenia saginata*, proglottids of, *170*
eggs of, *171*

*Taenia solium*
cysticercus, *170*
eggs of, *171*
proglottids of, *171*
scolex of, *170*

Tapeworms; *see* Cestodes

Tease mount technique, *144*

Tinsdale agar, *49*

Tissue culture flasks, *177*

Tissue culture tubes for viral detection, *176*

Tissue processing, *17*

*Torulopsis (Candida) glabrata*, differential identification of, *115*

*Toxocara canis*, embryonated egg and egg with larvae of, *165*

*Toxoplasma gondii*
cyst of, in brain tissue, *154*
indirect fluorescent method for detecting antibodies to, *197*
trophozoites of, *154*

Transgrow bottle, *11*

Trematodes, *146, 167–169*

*Treponema pallidum*, microhemagglutination assay for detecting antibodies to, *198*
RPR test, *199*

*Trichinella spiralis*, larvae of, in muscle, *164*

*Trichomonas hominis*, trophozoite of, in feces, *151*

*Trichophyton mentagrophytes*
Christiansen urea agar slant for demonstrating urease production by, *136*
lactophenol cotton blue preparation of, *135*
on Sabouraud's dextrose agar, *135*

*Trichophyton rubrum*
Christiansen urea agar slant for demonstrating urease production by, *136*
lactophenol cotton blue preparation of, *136*
on Sabouraud's dextrose agar, *135*

*Trichophyton schoenleinii*
lactophenol cotton blue preparation of, *136*
on Sabouraud's dextrose agar, *136*

*Trichophyton tonsurans*
lactophenol cotton blue preparation of, *137*
nutritional test for, *138*
on Sabouraud's dextrose agar, *137*

*Trichophyton verrucosum*
lactophenol cotton blue preparations of, *138*
on Sabouraud's dextrose agar, *138*

*Trichophyton violaceum*
lactophenol cotton blue and calcofluor white preparations of, *139*
on Sabouraud's dextrose agar, *139*

*Trichuris trichiura*
adult male, *162*
egg of, in feces, *162*

Triple sugar iron agar
for Enterobacteriaceae, *62*
reactions to, *63*

*Trypanosoma brucei gambiense*, blood of, *160*

*Trypanosoma brucei rhodesiense*, blood of, *160*

*Trypanosoma cruzi*, trypanomastigote of, *159*

Trypanosomiasis, *159–160*

TSI slant
*Campylobacter jejuni* on, *80*
*Enterobacteriaceae* on, *62, 63*
*Erysipelothrix rhusiopathiae* on, *50*
*Pseudomonas aeruginosa*, *83*
*Shewanella putrefaciens*, *85*

Turbidity meter, *107*

**U**

Uni-N/F-Tek for identifying *Stenotrophomones (Xanthomonas) maltophilia*, *85*

*Ureaplasma*, antibody detection of, by microimmunofluorescence test, *106*

*Ureaplasma urealyticum*
colonies of, *105*
transmission electron microscopy of, *106*

Urease test, *61*
for *Bordetella*, *77*
for *Brucella*, *77*
for *Cryptococcus neoformans*, *116*
for *Enterobacteriaceae*, *61*
for *Trichophyton mentagrophytes*, *136*
for *Ureaplasma urealyticum*, *105*

**V**

Vaccinia virus, transmission electromicroscopy, *192*

Vancomycin
anaerobe resistance to, *90*
*Pediococcus* resistance to, *44*
*Peptostreptococcus magnus* resistance to, *92*

Vancomycin susceptibility test of *Pediococcus*, *44*

Varicella zoster virus, *183*
antibody detection of, *186*
cytopathic effect, *186*
shell vial of, fluorescent stain of, *186*
in skin lesions
direct fluorescent assay of, 186
hemotoxylin and eosin stain of, *185*

*Veillonelta*, identification of, *90*

Vials, shell, *177*

*Vibrio*, *72*

*Vibrio cholerae*
on sheep blood agar, *81*
on TCBS, *81*
on thiosulfate-citrate-bile salts-sucrose (TCBS), *81*

*Vibrio parahaemolyticus*
on sheep blood agar, *81*
on TCBS, *81*

Virology, *176–193*

Viruses; *see also* specific viruses
collection and transport of, *10, 11*
detection and identification of, *176–193*

VITEK system, *111*

VITEK yeast biochemical card, *145*

**W**

Waste disposal, 5

*Wuchereria bancrofti*, microfilariae of, *166*

# X

X and V strips, *Haemophilius influenzae* on, *75*

*Xanthomonas* (scc *Stenotrophomonas*)

Xylose-lysine-desoxycolate, Enterobacteriaceae on, *58*

# Y

Yeast
    form of, *25*
    *versus* parasites, in feces, *174*

Yeast cells, Gram stain of, *31*

*Yersinia enterocolitica*, characteristic reactions of, *66*
    in API 20 E strips, *70*

# Z

*Zygomycetes*, diagram of, *124*